BROKEN LIKE ME

An Insider's Toolkit for Mending Broken People

Joseph Reid

ISBN: 978-1-7370786-1-6

PRAISE FOR *BROKEN PEOPLE*

"In the nine years that I have known Joseph, he has always been someone that showed genuine care for others. Because he cares so deeply for others and their well-being, the Broken People page was created. This is a place that people with mental health issues, no matter race, gender, ethnicity, or faith come to care, encourage, uplift, and support one another, or just vent without judgement. Joseph created a safe place for this to happen. I am honored to be able to call this man a friend."

AJ Coburn. Lansing, MI.

"Joe Reid has faced mental health challenges from an early age. Instead of allowing his issues to limit his effectiveness, Joe turned his energy toward helping others. Broken People is an outgrowth of Joe's heartfelt desire to benefit others with his experience. Joe is an excellent example of turning your problems into possibilities. What started as an online support group is turning into a support network for people with hurts, challenges, and fears. Joe demonstrates care and wisdom in managing Broken People. This book is just the next step in what I anticipate will be a series of helps for hurting, struggling people."

Dr. J. Paraiso. Murfreesboro, TN.

"Joseph Reid has been a major source of support for Broken People. Joe has lived through many tough journeys, making him one of the most caring and compassionate people I know. He is truly one of my closest friends. His peer support group, Broken People, has been a wonderful and major part of my life since 2018. I am actively involved and am privileged to work with Joe as part of his administrative team."

D. Cox. San Jacinto, CA.

"When Joseph first invited me to join Broken People, I did so never intending to participate. I was used to pretending publicly that everything was okay, until it wasn't. I went through a huge betrayal during a very difficult period of my life. Broken People and Joseph were there for me. They were the life preserver I needed to swim out of the abyss and back toward hope. This group and Joseph are Godsent, and I'm very thankful."

M. Couch. Detroit, MI.

"Joe's personal experience, persistent faith, and unique perspective give him profound insight into dealing with mental illness, whether it's in your own life or in the life of someone you love. This insight, along with his profound empathy for loved ones and strangers alike, will positively impact you and your ability to cope with whatever challenges you are facing."

C. Tiesma. Grand Rapids, MI.

"When I was heartbroken, I was searching for the broken online. So I joined Broken People. It's more than just a group full of heartbroken teenagers. It's a place full of people to help you, who have experiences like you do and care. It makes me feel good to go to people who understand and help and to also be helpful to other people who need it. It's like a family. A better family. If you have no one, you have someone ... if you don't have a therapist, even though we all live f@#$%oing far away from each other, it helps. Broken People is there."

C. Celice. Strausberg, Germany.

"With Broken People, Joe has tapped into something both simple and profound - our shared humanity. It is quite remarkable what can happen when people find a safe space to share their struggles. People feel less like they are alone, and more like they can press on. That's what has happened in Broken People."

D. Roede. Grand Rapids, MI.

For more about Broken People,
visit http://www.broken-people.org

If you'd like a downloadable, free workbook
that goes along with this book,
go to my website:

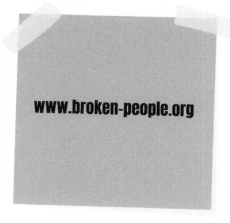

www.broken-people.org

Click on "contact us" in the menu,
and then enter your information.
In the comment section, just type

"I'd like the free workbook."

To my wife, Melissa. Shmily.

TABLE OF CONTENTS

Introduction

The First Tool

The Second Tool

The Third Tool

Introduction

"If you want to change the world,
pick up a pen and write."

Martin Luther

A NOTE FROM
THE AUTHOR'S DAUGHTER

Here is why mental illness makes me mad: oftentimes it is rooted in what is not real. Don't get me wrong, chemical imbalances are real, emotions are real, traumatizing events are real. But emotions that come from mental illness are sometimes the effects of invalid thinking. It took me several months to sit down in front of my computer and write about my experience growing up with my dad's mental illness. I've never had access to my dad's mind- the thoughts that kept him awake at night were unknown to me as a child. His hospitalizations came as a shock to me. When my mom told me she found a picture he drew of himself with a gun in his mouth, I was shocked. My memories of my dad have little to do with his mental illness and everything to do with how he was completely involved in my life, not afraid to embarrass himself for his kids, a serving husband, and a friend to the corners of society. I thank God that I remember my dad the way that I do, and that what my dad thought about himself—what he thinks about himself—is not true. If I were to remember my dad the way that he remembers himself, that would mean that mental illness wins. I get it now, Dad, I do. Not because you are any less than all you should be, but because I battle the thoughts too. If all you think about me is true, then you should know that your thoughts are lying to you. The lies only win when they are hidden, but I have seen you expose them over and over again and create community. I couldn't be prouder of who you are and the work that you are doing.

Hannah Reid

I'M BROKEN TOO

In 2002, I spent two weeks in a psychiatric hospital in West Michigan. My life was a mess. I'd regularly beat myself in the head with my fists, draw pictures of—and fantasize about—trying to kill myself, and write the most awful things about myself in my journal. I was at a point where I was scared to die, but I was convinced it was the only option. Ridiculous? Sure, but when you don't have the mental tools to know how to handle overwhelming frustration and depression, this is where your mind lands. That's when you resort to some pretty unique and hurtful coping mechanisms.

My wife saw what was going on. She saw how kind I was to other people while I abused and insulted myself in the shadows of our home. So she gave me a choice: check myself into the mental hospital voluntarily or she would call the police to come take me in. I did not like my options. The psych. hospital was for crazy people. I couldn't understand why she was doing this to me, or see that my wife was loving me the best way she knew how, by telling me truths I didn't want to hear. Please pay close attention when those who love you are telling you things you don't want to hear, especially during an emotional crisis. Find those people. Trust those people. It's in them that you will find the greatest of support.

And if you have trouble finding these people, keep reading. Help is on the way!

So, yeah, I went to the hospital. I stayed busy my first few days there with homework from a ministry school I was attending, while also trying to be helpful to the hospital staff. I felt like I didn't belong on "that side" of the glass. A few patients actually thought I worked there and would come to me for help. After a stern talking to from the therapist and my wife (an unfair tag team if ever there was one), I relinquished control of my books and stopped trying to be so helpful to other people. Only then did I begin the long process of learning to take care of me.

At this point, the psychiatrist decided I needed medication to help me settle down to a place where I could begin to heal. Seven days of my life were lost because of the medications I was given. I had no idea what was going on at the time, and I still have no memory of it to this day. Meds seemed to be the go-to method for dealing with people in my situation in those days. I knew even then, with my limited understanding of mental illness, that this method was missing a huge component. In fact, I had a pretty good idea that they were doing more harm than good—and, I wasn't too far off.

A lot happened during this hospitalization that messed with my head. I woke up one night to find a half-naked woman standing next to my bed, staring down at me. Another time, in between the patient checks that happened every fifteen minutes, two patients went and had sex in one of the showers.

Each room had two beds, so I had several roommates during my stay as people came and went. One was a male sex worker that had been admitted after mutilating his arm with a razor blade. I could see muscle and tendons when they brought him in on his first night. He didn't have a change of clothes—and openly admired my underwear, so I gave him a few pairs. It was the least I could do for him.

It wasn't all bad. Patients were generous sometimes. One older gentleman had a significant collection of firearm magazines, and he let me borrow a few. Just a little light reading to pass the time at a mental hospital, right?

One experience in particular really rattled my cage and left me traumatized for years to come. It started with a male patient who was wandering the halls at night. He would go into people's rooms and sit on their beds, naked. This creeped everyone out, so we told the staff about it. They warned him that this was not "acceptable behavior," but he didn't stop. He'd wander into a room, drop his drawers, and sit on a bed. Stand up. Pants up. Go to another room, rinse and repeat.

Finally, the staff had enough. One night—just a few days before I was discharged—this guy was switching rooms, and two staff members tried to corral him into the "time out room." (This was a locked room behind the staff desk with padded walls and a small access window for the inhabitant to receive food.) He wasn't having it. So many beds to sit on, so little time, I guess. As they reached for him to guide him toward his intended destination, he became aggressive. It started with some shoving. He wasn't going to let anyone put their hands on him. When it was clear that he was not going to go easily, they tried to subdue him with some type of nurse-jitsu. Somehow, all three of them ended up on the floor. They were right outside the door to my room, and I was pleading with the patient to just lay still. The female staff member yelled for me to get back into my room and close the door. Yes, ma'am! You don't have to tell me twice.

At that point I was shaking with fear, and I braced my body against the door to prevent the guy from getting in if he got away from the staff. Then I heard the female staff member warn her colleague to watch his hand because it appeared the patient was trying to bite it. The shouting grew louder until I heard the male attendant scream to the female that his finger was in the guy's mouth and that he was biting down. The patient must have bitten hard because then I heard screams, followed by a very loud, "He just bit off my finger!" As the female yelled for ice in a cup, the patient spit the finger out with a *thwap* right in front of my door. Still shaking, I yelled through my door, "Just drug the guy!" I could hear another member of the staff yelling into the phone to a 911 dispatcher.

The two attendants still held on to the patient despite one losing a finger, but at this point they were pleading for help from anyone. I heard another larger patient, my roommate at the time, go over to help hold the man down while they waited for the police to arrive. I stood frozen in fear for what seemed like an eternity, hand tightly clasped on the doorknob, foot braced against the door, waiting to hear the precious sounds of sirens in the distance. Cracking the door and braving a glance, I saw two officers rush into the hallway outside my room, stick their foot on the patient's back, and say three words that will be burned into my memory for all time: "This is over!" It was such a sweet sound. Such sweet relief!

So, yeah, the place felt a little out of control. With that said, I was just beginning to realize that I was one broken person in a world full of broken people. The naked lady standing next to my bed, the patients having sex in the shower, the guy with the cut up arm, the gentleman with the gun magazines, and the man that bit off the worker's finger… all hurting, broken people. Each one of them, all of us, deserve respect and need help. We are in this together.

Honesty is the best policy. I'm not sure who coined that phrase, but I think it's a good one. But, to be honest, honesty has been a battle I never knew was so connected to my mental illness. As you read earlier, I didn't uncover my mental illness until adulthood—I was about twenty-four at the time of my first hospitalization—and by then,

I had grown accustomed to lying in order to get what I wanted. I would lie to my friends because I believed that the person I was, wasn't good enough for them. In my high school Bible class, I made up a story that I was dying so that everyone would give me the attention I so, so, so longed for. How messed up is that? I literally lied in Bible class because I wanted everyone to gather around and pray for me.

Without a doubt, my choices made matters worse. I was reinforcing unhealthy and unsustainable life habits that I would later have to unlearn. To top it off, I really did love God, which led to a ton of guilt for my hypocritical behavior. I felt like such a fraud. I wore my religious faith like a badge of superiority. And yet, I felt completely inferior to everyone else. Dishonesty was a drug, and I was hooked. Why? Because it worked, at least in the short run. That's what makes addictions so appealing: they work. Unfortunately, addictions also hurt us and the ones we love. I had a sickness, and no one—myself included—understood the symptoms.

It wasn't until I adopted the policy of honesty and vulnerability that I was able to head down the healing path, away from mental illness and the need for external validation, and finally, toward recovery. It was also because of this significant choice that I found others who battled mental illnesses like I did. I was uncovering a strange new world where people thought and saw things the way I did. I'm really excited to share my story with you. I'm even more excited to tell you about some of the things I've learned and how I've applied them to my life. Thank you for giving me this opportunity.

So, yeah, I've learned a few things over the past twenty years. I've paid attention to my therapist, doctors, and wife, read dozens of books, and drank countless cups of chocolate milk. The result is a much healthier and happier life AND this book that I am writing for you.

*You*TILIZATION

Before we dig into the tools I've got for you, I'd like to introduce you to an idea: *You*tilization. *You*tilizing is a term I use to describe what happens when I hear or learn something new and adapt it to reflect who I am or the way I do things, making that thing or idea more reflective of who I am. This is one key component I want you to keep in the forefront of your mind as you read this book. The information in this book is great, but what will make it even better, is if you *You*tilize it. I've read books where the author says to dot the "i's" and cross the "t's" the way they do. This is usually followed by some sort of guarantee that your situation will turn out just like theirs. Hogwash. Just plain silliness. Here's what I want you to do with this book (and any future books you read on personal development): adapt them to fit your life…*You*tilize them. Don't worry if you're not sure how to do this yet, I've got some helpful tips throughout this book, so read on, reader!

Let's look at this from a musical perspective. Different songs have different melodies that make them unique, excellent, and beautiful. If you try to copy the melody of someone else's song, it becomes an imitation (or a really cool remix). A clone. That's not the life I want for you. Make your own music! That's why

*You*tilization is important. I want you to *You*tilize the tools in this book in a way that only you can. Take ownership of each tool I present and adapt it to your life. Each section will end with a *You*tilization challenge to help get you thinking and active in this process. Give these challenges some serious thought. Take it slow. I've tried to keep each section short so that you can read them in one sitting. After you've read it, take a look at the *You*tilization section and give it some thought.

Let me quickly tell you about Broken People, the international mental health support group that I lead. The idea behind the name is simple. When I am at my lowest point, feeling the most defeated and depressed, the most common thought that comes to mind is "I'm broken." So in an effort to find more people like me and draw them to the group, I named it Broken People. With that said, I think everyone has been—or is—broken to one degree or another. We all need help at some point to bring ourselves back together. That's what I'm doing with Broken People.

One last, very important thing: This book was not written by a mental health expert, so don't substitute it for receiving care from a doctor, therapist, or trained mental health professional. And please do not substitute this book for medication. The pages are much more difficult to digest and may lead to constipation. Instead, take your meds as prescribed.

*You*tilization

*You*tilization is already something each of us do every day without giving much thought to it. We find a way to do our job, clean our home, and cook our food that works *you*niquely for us. To someone else, our way may seem complicated or even a bit extreme, but it is our way, and a way we are comfortable with. As you go through your day, pay attention to the *you*nique way you do certain tasks.

One of the things I've really learned to embrace through loads of therapy is to accept the way I have adapted my life to meet certain challenges. Maybe you've heard the saying, "necessity is the mother of invention?" That definitely applies to people with a mental illness. Once you see the *you*niqueness of how you do certain things, write about it in your journal, and then pat yourself on the back!

ABOUT GOD

I've got a remarkable four foot by six foot painting of the Grand Rapids, Michigan skyline hanging on my living room wall that my daughter painted for my forty-fourth birthday. I've been wanting something like it for a while but never expected one to be made specifically for me. She's never done anything like this before, and it turned out amazing! I didn't get it right on my birthday because of the global Covid-19 pandemic. The night we celebrated my birthday and she presented it to me was also the night that protests were happening all over the country in response to the murder of George Floyd.

Prejudice is ugly, isn't it? And it comes in so many shapes and sizes. That night in my city, thousands of people from all walks of life got together to peacefully protest the continued presence of racism in our country. Toward the end of the night, a lot of damage had been done to our downtown district. It was a mess of graffiti, broken glass, and trash.

Someone created a Facebook event to clean up the damage the next day. Just like the majority of the previous days' protests, it was a wonderful expression of community and solidarity. I decided to go, but I knew that by the time I was able to get up and head out after a long shift the night before, most of the cleanup would be done. Hundreds of people showed up with brooms and dustpans. Restaurant owners came and handed out free food. Church congregations came and sang songs of hope. I went with my story, some wristbands from my support group, and my daughter's painting.

When I got there, just as I'd thought, most of the cleanup was completed. I took my painting to the busiest area of the city, Rosa Parks' Circle—where there is a small outdoor amphitheater, and stood in front of the stage. Right in the center. It was one of the most uncomfortable things I'd ever done. I just stood there. And, I had no idea what I was going to do next. That was as far as I planned up to that point. As I stood there, staring out at all the people loving each other and at the buildings towering all around me, I noticed something: my painting was all wrong. I still thought it was amazing, but it didn't look at all like the actual skyline. My daughter had taken many of the beautiful buildings from all over our city and brought them together to create one masterpiece. When all these structures came together in this work of art, I was left with this magnificent act of love hanging on my wall that I will cherish forever.

Buildings are stuck. They're not going anywhere. But an artist, a creator, my daughter, took these immovable objects and brought them together. Wouldn't it be beautiful if that would happen for us? Then it struck me that that was what these protests were all about: Trying to change things that seem stuck in the fabric of our society. Wouldn't it be incredible if we could get people, systems, and organizations unstuck from their prejudices and find unity and community with people who are not like us?

It seems to me that if there is a God who is the great artist and creator of all things, that he would be thoroughly vested in getting his creation unstuck from personal prejudice. I think he is. But, sadly, many of those who claim to be his followers are guilty of some of the worst, most destructive prejudices this world has ever experienced. I am also guilty of propagating prejudices because of my own ignorance. As far back as I can remember, I have tried to follow the ways of Jesus. Much of that time "following Jesus" was spent separating myself from others. I built walls to protect myself from the "sin and depravity" of the world. This is one of those behaviors I've been working diligently to unlearn.

God plays a big part in the story of my personal and emotional healing, and because of that, I bring him up throughout the book. I know that you've probably been hurt by people like me, and for this I am so, so sorry. It is my firm belief that this is the result not of prejudicial design or lack of interest on God's part, but of the prejudices of a group of people who are trying to assume God's role. Oddly, or not so oddly, enough, this is one of the largest accusations against Lucifer and why he was cast out of God's presence. I'm just spit-balling here, but it's probably not a good idea to take cues from the Prince of Darkness.

This book is all about helping people with their mental illness. I know that many "so-called" churches have really hurt people who fall into this category by judging, ignoring, minimizing, or demonizing their struggle. But please know that there are people who are trying to follow Jesus and are turning a significant corner. There is a very intentional and concerted effort to try to obliterate our prejudices, and so many of us are daily seeking God's help to do so.

If you have been hurt by people who claim to love God and to be doing His will, please give me just a little bit of leeway. I'm not writing this book to change your mind about religion or to justify what has been done to you. So much stuff that has been done throughout history in the name of God is just a load of crap. We live in such a broken world, full of broken people. When I talk about God here, I am sharing with you stuff that has been helpful to me. That's all. It's been a very long and hard personal journey. I am learning to let my walls down and to love like Jesus loved.

*You*tilization

Do you think you are better than other people? I know this is not something that anyone would want to admit, but I think it is something all of us feel at some point or another. In the previous chapter, you read that *you*tilization is taking an idea or activity and making it work for you. Have you ever been in a relationship where someone is absolutely convinced you are doing something wrong, when in fact you are just doing something differently than the way they do it?

Think about your least favorite genre of music. Say it out loud. Now, here is your challenge: Listen to at least two songs from that genre before you read the next chapter, then ask yourself, "What do I think about the type of people who listen to this music?" Despite the fact that you really don't enjoy this type of music, some people do. It is *good music* to someone. That's all for this challenge. Just remember that just because you don't like or agree with something, doesn't mean that it is bad or wrong.

55 - 5: SUCCESS

We won the game 55-5. It was the last game of the year and a really big deal for me. It was my first year playing organized sports. I was a forward on the Kinyon Elementary Roadrunner's sixth grade basketball team. I'd been cut from the basketball team the previous year because my grades were too low, so this was pretty important to me. The coach was an animated guy, jumping around, yelling, and waving his hands, as coaches do. My grandparents were there: Grandpa Roscoe with his VHS camcorder, and Grandma with her Cinnamon Trident. My parents were there: Mom, with her yellow and blue pom poms, Dad, just hoping I'd do my best, and my brothers, who were either there because they were forced to be or because they'd been bribed with a few dollars for the concession stand. The game was being recorded. This was serious. It felt like my entire future was on the line.

I usually only played about two minutes of a twenty-four-minute game which gives you some idea of how good I was. I was such a motivated kid, with just a little skill, and even less confidence. This story is an example of one of my earliest recollections of batting my mental illness. I was beginning to experience a part of me that seemed somehow broken. I was so convinced that if I tried hard enough, I'd be able to go pro one day, but I was constantly faced with the knowledge that I was one of the worst players on the team. I was a boy who was stuck in his imagination.

When that last game was over, I remember that our team got this large and impressive trophy proclaiming our dominance on the hard wood. The trophy was passed around, and all the cool kids got to hold it. The good players, the ones with all the playing time, points,

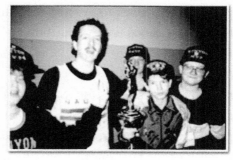

and prestige, for sure got their time in. I just wanted out of there. I donned my 1980s rayon blue, track-style jacket, grabbed my gym bag, and headed for the door. I was a loser. I didn't contribute to this game. I played two minutes in a game that was literally won with our third basket. My team succeeded. I know I should've felt like a part of that success, but I didn't. On my way out of the gym, my mom got the coach and a few team members together for a picture of me with the trophy. I was "smiling", surrounded by my teammates. But if you take a look, maybe you can you see the struggle behind that smile. It's there. I didn't like myself. I didn't like my life.

Success is a hard topic, right? How often have you felt that you are—and always will be—a failure? I can't write a book about mental health and not address this "success" issue. People with a mental illness are already hard enough on themselves, never feeling good enough, never feeling like they measure up. Success is one of those subjects that sends me into a near crushing panic attack.

Is it just me, or does success seem like a bad word sometimes? That's weird, right, because the word literally means, "a favorable or desired outcome[1]." But there are two sides to every coin, and this coin certainly has its ugly side. When you think about success, which I'd really like you to do as you read this section, consider the internal and external expectations. I saw a meme recently that said, "The planet does not need more successful people. The planet desperately needs more peacemakers, healers, restorers, storytellers, and lovers of all kinds." This quote seems to suggest that there is something wrong with success. But why?

Consider a few examples of why success may get a bad rap:

First, there are times when it seems necessary for people to fail in order for someone else to succeed. This is why competitiveness is being frowned upon in our schools these days. In a competitive game, someone wins and someone loses, which is equated with success and failure. When people lose, it doesn't feel good. When people fail it sucks, right?

Second, success is often associated with wealth. There is a general feeling, just like in a competition, that the rich are winning and the poor are losing. This is a big deal because it seems like the financial aspect of our success is rigged... and maybe it is? As I alluded to in the previous chapter, prejudices of all sorts exist, and this is no exception. Those who are not rich may think that the wealthy are manipulating the system to take advantage of everyone else, while the rich may think that those who are not are lazy and unintelligent. This is the kind of success I think the meme above speaks of. It's one that is based on some pretty big assumptions about financially successful people. I agree that the world needs fewer people consumed with money and attaining material things, but this isn't the only kind of success. Success is impartial, meaning that it doesn't matter what the thing is that someone is doing. It is a label we give to experiences and people when a goal has been achieved.

Here is one last example of why success seems to have a negative connotation. Some people, when they succeed, appear to be so consumed with their success that it seems like they don't give a rip about anyone else. They give the impression that they made it to where they are all by themselves. And if they do acknowledge others that have helped along the way, it is often insincere, fake, and forced.

Success is all around us, and we probably experience it more than we realize. It has been helpful for me to acknowledge this as I battle my depression. Did you make it to work on time today? If you were late, did you make it in at all? If not, were you sick and called in? If you accomplished any one of the aforementioned tasks today, you were successful at something. And, if none of those situations applies to you, you can at least say you were successful at reading this entire paragraph. Good job!

I'd like to suggest that success is not only important, but vital, for our mental health. In fact, our very existence depends upon success. We depend on the success of farmers to get food to the grocery stores. We depend on the success of our doctors and scientists to make specific medications to help with our symptoms. We depend on water treatment plants to succeed at filtering out harmful bacteria. Humanity's entire existence depends upon success.

One progressive step toward being a successful person is finding out what success means to you. We could read every religious text, all the self-help books, and listen to every single motivational speaker to have ever graced this planet with their perfectly manicured nails and wavy hair, and still be left wanting if *we* don't have some idea of what success means to us. Figuring this out can be extremely tricky, right? But why!? Pastors and priests, authors, those glamorous motivational speakers, our bosses, spouses, friends, and mothers-in-law all have their own opinions of what true success is. If we don't define what it means to us, we will be constantly chasing the ever-changing view of success that other people have around us. Don't despair if you have no idea where to begin. I'm here to help.

Have you ever heard someone say," Success is a journey, not a destination?" It sounds great, doesn't it? But no matter how hard I try to believe it—and believe me I've tried—the journey either feels unimportant, really boring, or like excruciatingly hard work. That's how I felt at that final game of the season when I spent most of the time on the bench—very, very unimportant and bored. I would like to offer an alternative to the quote above and say that success is both a journey AND a destination.

Consider the timeline of an experience. At the beginning of the timeline is a decision: the establishment of a personal goal, desired change, etc.

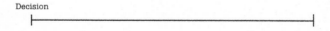

Where on this timeline would you place success?

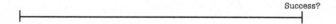

I've always put success at the end of the timeline. It's the idea that we've succeeded when we've accomplished something we set out to do. It might be winning first prize in an art competition, graduating with a 4.0, or scoring the game winning point in the final game of the season (which is impossible to do when you're sitting on the bench for most of the game, I might add … come on, coach!). But this way of thinking creates a disturbing problem. Is there only one success story in an art competition? Is there only success for those who set out to reach a certain grade and attain it? Is the only successful person in a basketball game the one who scores the final point to break the tie? If not, is this failure? As you read through this book, I hope you'll see that I've challenged the perception that success is either a journey OR a destination. Instead, I hope to motivate you to discover success in every part of an experience.

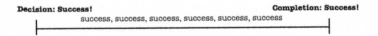

Decision: Success!   Completion: Success!
success, success, success, success, success, success

I want you to realize that you are succeeding when you start something, when you continue it, when you fall or fail, when you start again, and when you finish. Success awaits us in every aspect of a journey but oftentimes goes unseen because emotions and expectations get in the way.

Wait … Did I just say there is success when we fail? Most certainly. There is no success without failure. It's a package deal. In fact, the more we allow ourselves to fail, the more often we succeed. Why? Because there is no greater teacher than failure. But we need to stop hiding our failures as if they are something to be ashamed of and begin the process of learning to accept and, more importantly, celebrate them.

This may be a significant paradigm shift for you, and maybe you're wondering if it lessens the meaningfulness of success? "Doesn't this mean that everyone is a success?" Not entirely, but you're catching on! This notion of success does not fall into the "everyone is a winner" category. There is an important distinction: winning first place in something and success are not the same thing.

The only way to truly not succeed is to give up. But even then, quitting may be a really great choice depending on the circumstances. If you, for example, sought to rob a bank; you plan, research, study, create maps, and put together the ideal team. But then you, as an act of conscience, abort the mission. You quit. You didn't succeed at robbing the bank. But you did succeed at not going to jail and not scaring the crap out of a bunch of bank employees and customers. Good choice by the way!

One final note about success: We all want to have a fulfilled life. If we don't feel fulfilled, something's gotta give. You and I are unique, and how we live and what we enjoy is going to reflect that uniqueness. Consider a song. Our lives have a beginning, a middle, and an end. The Beetles song "A Hard Day's Night" starts quickly with "It's been a hard day's night, and I've been working like a dog (Lennon & McCartney, 1964)." What if the song ended there? What's so great about working hard all night? But the song ends with, "You know I feel alright." Whew! We worked hard, and we feel good.

BUT ... what if those were the only parts we ever heard—just the beginning and end lines? Well, we'd never have found out that "When I'm home everything seems to be right. When I'm home feeling you holding me tight." Our lives consist of a beginning, middle, and an end. We need all three. We don't really have a choice in the matter. We don't get to choose our beginning, and we have very little say about our ending, but there is a beautiful in-between, combined with the beginning and end, that makes our lives complete. Just like "A Hard Day's Night," each strum, each note played, all of it, is success. Each decision you make, each path you take, I'll be watching you .... oh wait, different song. Each decision you and I make, each path we take, it's all part of this song that is our life. We can't get rid of the middle, so we do the best we can with what we have. This book is a great way to help you get there.

Are you dealing with difficult life stuff? Maybe you don't feel like the beautiful in-between is all that beautiful. This book is for you! I understand what you're going through. I understand the constant feeling of never being good enough, of continually feeling like a failure. I hope to inspire you to see life in a fresh, new way and to help you become aware and mindful of your personal awesomeness! You and I see our failures and shortcomings quite clearly, but I'm learning—and hope to encourage and enable you to as well—to see the successes along this journey, and to celebrate them in a fulfilling way.

*You*tilization

I've found that I'm naturally drawn to remember the things I screw up. These are the things I've forgotten to do, haven't done very well, or the stuff I've decided not to do at all. It's much harder for me to look back and see what I have succeeded at. And it certainly isn't easy to look back and label my failures as a sort of success.

Last night as I was preparing this section, I accidentally sent a text to my daughter that was meant for my wife, asking her, "What are some of the successes in my life?" She sent me back a list of twenty things in a very short time. That's your challenge today. Text at least two loved ones and ask them the same question: "What are some of the successes in my life?" I think and hope that you may be a little surprised at what you receive back.

The
First Tool

Imagine an old, rusty, red toolbox, like the kind that your parents or grandparents had back in the day. We're going to dig into it and explore different tools you and I can use to help us along in our mental health journey. The first tool we're going to look at is the most important of them all—is there a "most important tool of them all?" you ask. Absolutely. So, let's see here. There's a hammer on top, that's not it. It's big, heavy, and powerful though, but we'll get to that later. A box of nails is sitting in the corner. Nope, it's not those either. Screwdriver, another screwdriver, utility knife, and a Lord of the Rings Lego figure. How did that get in here? There it is! Our first—and the most important—tool. I love this thing! It's a measuring tape.

A measuring tape helps us measure distance, but there are many other tools used to measure things, like a scale, thermometer, clock, speedometer, measuring cups, and a calendar, to name a few. Measuring is a normal function of our day. It's one of the most important things humans have learned to do, often without even thinking about it. We measure when we check the time, do our laundry, cook, fill our gas tank, or play a game. We use this skill all the time. Measurement has the potential to save and transform lives. Despite the undeniable importance of this one tool, it has been horribly neglected by the mental health community. Let me explain why and what we can do about it.

WHY DO WE NEED A
MENTAL HEALTH SCALE

I am blessed with incredible kids. They are thoughtful and sincere human beings. But, just like any human being, they can do incredibly stupid stuff sometimes. For a while, when my youngest daughter first started driving, I'd get a call every other week or so that she ran out of gas. I tried to remind her that the gas gauge was there to help her keep that from happening. Eventually she did learn, and it's been a couple years since I've gotten the "Dad, I'm out of gas" call. I did, however, get a "Dad, my car is making a funny noise. My oil light is on. Should I keep driving?" call late one night not too long ago. After meeting up with my very sweet, very intelligent, but sometimes forgetful daughter, I reminded her that cars need oil. My daughter learned that measuring incorrectly, or forgetting to measure at all, can be a very costly mistake.

We measure time to avoid being late. We don't overload our washing machines because we want our laundry to get clean without breaking it. We've got lots of measuring tools that make life a bit easier. Measuring spoons, gas gauges, scales, and on and on. All sorts of measurements go into building a skyscraper. We calculate distance when throwing a pass, and adjust the force of the throw, because we want to win a game. Our car measures miles with the odometer so that we don't run out of gas. And, as my daughter learned, there is a dipstick that helps measure oil and avoiding that measurement is quite expensive. Measurement always involves a "because" linked with some form of communication. Measurement keeps us safe, keeps us moving, and creates boundaries for us to live in and function. But it is pretty useless if we don't do it or communicate it.

Before I get any further into the importance of measuring, I want to address why there is a need for any type of mental health scale in the first place: When you struggle with mental illness, it can be tough for people to understand what you are dealing with, especially those you've never dealt with before or people who are close with someone who has a mental illness. Being able to communicate how you're feeling to your loved ones, medical professionals, and law enforcement, can literally be a matter of life or death. Using a scale like the one I am going to teach you here, will help you communicate better, track your emotional fluctuations—either up or down, and help your loved ones respond appropriately if you're emotionally slipping or track and celebrate when you are doing well. So, without further ado, here is the tool, aptly called the Mental Health Scale (MHS). My friends also refer to this as The Joe Scale because, well … I made it. This thing is so powerful! It enables you to understand where you are, effectively communicate it, and then take the necessary steps to stay healthy and be safe. It also gives you a super simple way to deal with the dreaded "How are you?" question.

*You*tilization

You are getting ready to learn how to communicate how you're doing with loved ones in a very simple and clear way. But communication is only as good as the person's willingness to share. Take a few minutes to make a mental note, or to jot down in your journal, a few people in your life that you'd trust you could give an honest answer to in any circumstance. Whether feeling good or bad, you can see yourself not holding back or trying to gloss over how you are doing because you know they genuinely care. And before you think that you may be tiring these people out with your sad story constantly, think about how you feel about them. Do they exhaust you when they share their struggles? I doubt it. No. Because you love them and want to know when and how to love them more. That's what this tool does. It lets your trusted community of support and loved ones know exactly how you are doing and can give them some insight about how they may be able to help you get moving in the right direction.

HOW ARE YOU?

I consider myself a kind, Christian, non-violent kind of guy, but if the phrase "How are you?" was a person, I would punch them in the nose. I mean a full force, close fisted, "give it all I've got" kind of punch. So yeah, I am not a fan.

How are you even supposed to answer a question like that? Are you supposed to say anything? Do you respond with a polite greeting, ask a similar question in return, or just ignore it entirely? I guess it depends on who's asking and what their relationship is to you, doesn't it? Here are a few other things to consider: Where are you when they ask? Are they walking quickly or slowly? Are they asking you or someone else standing close by? Are they wearing a green shirt? Oh, and did you check the barometric pressure? You gotta check that too! I feel like I go through an emotional calculus equation every time I am posed with the "How are you?" question. Why, you ask? Well, despite the fact that I'm not even sure it's an actual question, you still have to consider how thorough or truthful of an answer to give. And the truth is, it's just not that simple of a question to answer. See if you can relate to any of these feelings, thoughts, and/or responses I commonly have to the question: "Joe, how are you?"

−I feel like crap. Do I tell them I feel like crap? Do they even want to know? Is this one of those tricky rhetorical questions my therapist warned me about? I don't want to lie to them. I don't want them to think that I think they don't care. Do I need to validate them because they took the time to check in on me? If this person isn't someone I trust to dump my sorry stories on, do I risk being honest and open up the potential for a longer conversation with someone I'd rather not take time to talk to about my problems? Do they even have enough time as they're walking by to hear my answer? "I'm great!"

−I feel like crap and since you asked, I am going to tell you and see how you respond. This should be fun. "I feel like crap, how are you?"

−I feel like crap, and I am going to answer you honestly to scare you away without asking the question in return to avoid further interaction. "Awful, today sucks."

−I feel like crap and am so beside myself with emotion that I am going to grunt in your direction while looking down because I don't have the emotional energy to say or do anything else. "Grunt."

−Today is a hard day, I feel like crap, and I want to kill myself. But telling you would probably create a lot of drama that I don't want to deal with while wanting to kill myself. "I'm fine."

−I feel great, but I kind of feel guilty for feeling great because I usually feel like crap, and I know so many people around me feel like crap too. "I'm fine."

Those are some heavy emotions, right? But for some reason, I think you get it. And if you don't, if you're reading this and you yourself or someone you are close to does not have a mental illness, you may be a little shocked or put off by the abrupt heaviness of some of the thoughts I deal with on a daily basis. Welcome to my world and the wonderful world of the mentally ill.

Listen, I get it. It's not unmannerly for people to ask questions they don't intend to have answered. In fact, in our culture, asking someone how they are doing is a casual and polite greeting. It's not something meant to offend or annoy anyone. But for people with social anxiety, this isn't easy to understand. That's why I am very intentional about who I ask this question to. I won't ask someone how they're doing if I'm too busy to listen to a sincere answer. I'm also very careful with my empathic boundaries and try to avoid asking someone when I don't think I'd be able to handle a negative answer. Why? I have a history of burying myself quite quickly and deeply under the hardest emotions of other people. This is where my mental illness and my beautiful gift of empathy cause great friction in my life. I feel very fortunate to have an awareness of suffering around me, because I truly care for people. But the burden of so much suffering also weighs me down.

As you go through the next few chapters and figure out how to use the Mental Health Scale, maybe give some time and thought to how you feel about the "How are you?" question. Let's begin with how the Mental Health Scale works.

*You*tilization

Answering the "How are you?" question is tricky. And it's not like you or I want to be rude about it. So for this exercise, set a timer for fifteen minutes and come up with three or more responses to the "How are you?" question. Let these be your intentional replies so that it's no longer a tough battle about how to answer. Also, for at least one reply, try to be creative ... funny even. Check out the internet for unique replies to this question. Have some fun with it, and who knows, you may even make the person asking's day as well.

I like what I found on this website:

www.pairedlife.com/etiquette/Funny-and-Witty-Responses-to-the-Question-How-Are-You.

HOW IT WORKS

In 1999, a rocket launched into outer space was meant to orbit Mars to do scientific research and study the weather, then report back to Earth. Prior to taking orbit around Mars, communication was lost with the spacecraft. It is believed to have burned up in Mars' atmosphere. Why did this happen? Well, the simple answer is that there was a measuring error. The not so simple answer, however, will be revealed a little later and will hopefully convince you that you should use the Mental Health Scale for your mental health needs.

In the introduction to this unit, when I said that the mental health community has neglected this very important tool, this is what I meant: When we fail to measure things accurately, it makes it very difficult to communicate with people and solve problems. This group of chapters is all about getting everyone on the same page when evaluating someone's mental health because when things are measured poorly, inconsistently, or not at all, they have a tendency to go horribly wrong or fall apart. The Mental Health Scale is designed to be a universal scale for:

- people suffering with a mental illness,
- loved ones,

- organizations,

- and professionals such as law enforcement, therapists, doctors, etc.

We need it to create a common understanding of a person's mental health condition. While the scale is subjective, there are certain indicators (discussed a bit later) to help guide the user to a more accurate number.

The most common scale I've seen and used when going to meet with my therapist is the 1-10 scale, which can be confusing for so many reasons. One serious problem with any scale of this kind is knowing which direction it's going. Just this morning, while researching mental health scales, I ran across one that has the number one as doing very well and the ten as really bad (I will refer to this type as the Positive One Scale). Last night, someone shared a scale in the Broken People Facebook group where the reversal is true (the Positive Ten Scale). If you've spent any time with a therapist or psychiatrist, you're typically given a scale that works something like this: "Just tell me," they ask, "on a scale from one to ten, how are you feeling today?" Think about where you are emotionally right now. Referring to the Positive Ten Scale where ten is great and one is horrible, how would you answer this? Give it a number and write it in the box below.

Whether you pick two, five, or ten, you have to ask yourself what these numbers really mean. I always wonder, *Where is the line between feeling good and feeling bad on a scale from one to ten?* If ten is really good and one is really bad, where on the scale is the emotional equator? I'm a black and white kind of guy, so a five seems like the logical choice. It is the midpoint after all. This makes complete sense until I asked myself about the number four. According to this scale and how I perceive it, a four means I'm not doing so well. And, to be honest, a four really doesn't seem like all that bad of a number. In fact, to me, a four feels pretty darn good. Dealing with this internal frustration and confusion is another reason I decided to create the Mental Health Scale.

I'm usually not in the mood to give a big, long, honest answer to the "How are you?" question. When someone who truly cares about me and my situation asks me how I'm doing, I often feel like, "If I take my finger out of this hole in my emotional dam for just one second to answer you, the whole thing is going to burst and the destruction and resulting clean-up will be catastrophic." So then, how do I respond to a truly caring friend, professional, or family member in a way that will make sense to them when I feel like crap and don't have the energy or emotional fortitude to give a lengthy answer? That's another really great reason why I've developed this scale. It enables me to give a quick answer that communicates very clearly and succinctly how I am doing but requires little emotional effort and few words.

I can keep my finger in the dam and not risk anyone's life.

Let's get back to our missing orbiter. So, why did the Mars mission fail? When the rocket was designed, the builder, Lockheed Martin, installed software for the thruster system that used measurements in pounds of force. However, the software that was receiving navigational information from NASA read the data in the metric unit, so the failure happened because the two entities were basically speaking a different mathematical language. NASA was sending electronic messages for the craft to use specific amounts of thrust to position itself correctly, but the ship was receiving data and calculating in terms of pounds. Mental health professionals and the mentally ill need to start speaking the same language if we are going to beat these very complicated diseases. Imagine this tool in the hands of friends, loved ones, and caring professionals. This powerful communication tool, or at least something like it, I think could revolutionize how we understand and communicate pain and suffering, as well as success and happiness. And the Mental Health Scale, I believe, is the perfect tool. Just think how many emotional crashes we could avoid if everyone started to measure mental health in a universal way?

Here is how the scale works. Grab a piece of paper and a pen to get started. Don't worry. I'll wait.

. . .

. . .

. . .

Ok, good, you're back. Now draw a horizontal line. If you're using lined paper, draw the line from margin to margin. At the very center of the line, make a mark and write the number zero. Next, all the way to the right, write "+10," then all the way to the left, write "-10." Now go ahead and fill in the rest of the numbers in between while I go get a sandwich.

Turkey, Turkey, Cheese.

Did someone eat all the multigrain bread?

Oh, I just remembered I don't like sandwiches.

I'm back. Ok, so here's how it works. Start by asking yourself, "Self, how do you feel today?" If you feel good, your number will fall somewhere on the right side of the scale (the positive side). If you feel bad, it will fall on the left side (the negative side). For context, a +10 is the absolute best someone can feel, and a -10 is the worst possible feeling. A zero is that awful in-between where you're not feeling one way or the other. The days I am at a zero feel like I am teetering on an emotional precipice. I can't figure out how I feel, and so I find myself waiting for something to happen to tip me one way or the other. Those are my zero days. Just blah.

When you acknowledge where you are on the scale, that number is your Mental Health Number (MHN). At this very moment, my MHN is hovering around the -4.5 mark. Not good, right? Yeah, tell me about it!

Here are two additional numbers to be aware of: the Crisis Number and Manic Number. My family and friends know that if I ever hit a -6 or lower, I need to be taken immediately to the hospital. A -6 means that I have constant thoughts of suicide, mixed with a cycle of overwhelming hopelessness. It is my Crisis Number (CN).

There is another indicator on the scale that I also watch very closely. This is called the Manic Number (MN). Whenever I hit a +6, my MN, a big imaginary caution sign pops up in my head letting me know that it's possible I'm experiencing a manic episode. When that red flag goes up, I'm reminded to prepare myself for the potential of an emotional crash. It alerts me to ask the question, "Am I manic?"

Is it possible to hit a +6 and not be manic? Absolutely. This is why it's so important for us to enjoy the positive emotions and feelings we experience. Be present where you are: mind, body, and soul. I've learned to have positive coping skills at the ready should I experience an emotional avalanche, which usually follows manic episodes. The goal here is to avoid and/or prepare for a drastic drop in my MHN, while being mindful of, and hopefully enjoying, the good feelings in the moment. Whatever you do, don't allow the fear of having a manic episode steal the joy of a really high MHN and miss the awesomeness of having great feelings.

You may be wondering what a -10 looks like. A -10 means you are in the process of carrying out a suicide attempt. You've got the gun, the rope, the pills, whatever. The plan is set in motion. It's the worst possible situation.

I set up this scale to fit my needs a long time ago. But it is far more important and goes way beyond meeting the needs of just one person. When you are doing well, it adds to the overall health of your community. This strategy and tool is all about you taking everything you learn in therapy, support groups, and books (especially this book; wink, wink), and adapting it to your very own mental health strategy. The process of adaptation, which I explained in an earlier chapter, is called *You*tilization. *You*tilize this scale to fit your life.

Everyone is different. Not only do we have different strengths and weaknesses, but we also have different families, therapists, medications, jobs, and on and on. How does this play out? Maybe your Crisis Number is higher than mine, for example a -3 or -4. When you are feeling well, communicate that to your support network, walk them through each part of the MHS so they know what it all means. Then, hopefully, they will understand your situation and needs and be better equipped to know how to help should an emergency arise.

*You*tilization

You may have already guessed what exercise comes next. Tell two people you trust about the Mental Health Scale and how it works. Decide on—and then communicate—both your Crisis Number and Manic Number. Finally, let them know one or two things they could do to help you in each situation.

ADDITIONAL STUFF

You've heard me mention the word "manic" quite a few times now, but you may not know what it means. If you've never had a manic episode, it may be difficult for you to understand. There are two major types of manic episodes: manic and hypomanic. When someone is manic, they experience uncontrollable feelings of motivation and energy. This sometimes results in the person being hospitalized because their connection with the reality of their physical, intellectual, and emotional limitations and capabilities is often completely depleted (This is an example of Bipolar 1). A person who is hypomanic has many of the same symptoms as a person who is manic, but to a more manageable degree, thus not requiring hospitalization (an example of Bipolar 2). Here is a list of symptoms from Healthline.com to watch for:

- increased energy levels

- inability to relax

- decreased motivation to sleep

- unnatural increase in a person's self-esteem and confidence

- extreme fidgeting

- increased activity with new ideas and passions out of the blue

- doing too many things at once without the ability to finish them

- increased libido

- easily distracted

- decreased self-control

- impulsive behavior

But how do you know if you or someone you love is being manic or is just in a really good mood? Ask yourself or your loved one if they are sleeping enough. Have the emotions you have experienced been around for multiple days, or is it a mood that's unique for today? If they aren't getting enough sleep and have long instances of a euphoric type mood, it could indicate the presence of mania. It's really hard for anyone to diagnose someone as going through a manic episode, and suggesting to someone you care about that they may be manic can be problematic. You should always leave the heavy lifting when it comes to diagnosing and treating to the professionals. But it may be a good idea for you to lovingly encourage them to seek a professional's guidance if you suspect something's up.

Just this past week, I communicated back and forth with a friend whose MHN was dropping fast. It went from a -3 in the morning to a -5 in the afternoon. This is obviously not a good trajectory. The Mental Health Scale was useful because it helped my friend realize how bad her situation was and clearly communicate it with people who cared about her. From there, she was able to identify appropriate coping skills and ask for support from several friends until her situation improved.

What are coping skills? They are specific actions, kind of like emergency protocols, a person takes to deal with all sorts of emotional struggles. When applied, these skills are able to stall the downward trajectory of someone's MHN at the least, and possibly even move a person's emotional needle in the right direction—toward the positive side of the scale. Coping skills are temporary solutions to temporary crises.

At the end of the week, my friend messaged me to let me know she was up to a -1. Any movement in the literal right direction on the scale is fantastic and should be celebrated. A -1 is bad, right? Well, sort of… but it is a remarkable improvement from a -5. I quickly messaged her back acknowledging her progress and to celebrate her achievement! Acknowledging and celebrating what you or someone you care about has accomplished is crucial to the healing process. It's an absolute necessity for a healthy emotional lifestyle.

I use this scale for far more than just my mental health (which is why my wife and kids usually call it the Joe Scale). I've used it for everything from my wife's cooking to the state of the economy. This has been extremely helpful because my family has learned to understand how the scale works and even use it themselves on occasion.

One particular evening, my wife prepared an amazing meal and asked me to give it a rating on the Joe Scale. I told her it was an easy +7 or +8. Everyone at the table understood that a rating this high was extremely rare and deserved special attention—that is, until I kept talking. "Honey, this is so delicious! Did it come from a can?" In my defense, this was intended to be high praise, and would have been understood as such if it were my mother, father and brothers all seated around the table. The point here is that the more you use the Mental Health Scale/Joe Scale model, including for stuff other than just your mental health, the quicker and more comfortable you will become with how it works. And when you introduce and use it with others, you are reinforcing the principles of the scale and reminding them of its significance in your life.

If you are reading this book because you care about someone with a mental illness and want to understand their situation better, here is a brief list of steps you can take when they are struggling.

If your loved one comes to you and lets you know they've reached their crisis or manic number, it's important to:

- Completely focus on them. Be fully present. And if you can't, tell them and then be as supportive as you can.

- Assure them of your love.

- Listen to them. I can't stress this enough. Listen to their struggles.

- Prove to them that you have actually listened by repeating back what you heard. If you've gotten something wrong, or don't completely understand, this will help clear things up.

- Encourage them to seek appropriate professional care. If they have reached their crisis number, help them find a way to get to the nearest emergency room. If they've hit their manic number, ask them what coping skills they have to help them and/or what you can do for them.

*You*tilization

You've got a couple of people in your life that are learning the Mental Health Scale. That's great! This next challenge is to tell a few more. Teach it to your therapist, primary care physician, mom, dad, wife, husband, kids. Not only will this be helpful to you, but it will be a tool they can use in their lives as well.

The
Second Tool

We've taken a look at how measuring is a great way for us to begin improving our mental health because it lets us know where we are emotionally and what direction we need to be headed. The next couple of tools will help us get there. Let's head back to the tool box and see what other tools we can learn to use as we develop our mental health.

This next tool is heavy and can be a little intimidating. Despite its simplicity, you can do a lot with it. If you've tried to use it before and given up because it's too awkward, you don't feel coordinated enough, or maybe you've walked away from it in pain, you are not alone. I'm hoping you'll let me convince you to give it another shot. I've had some experience with it, and I think I can teach you a better, safer way to use it. The second tool we will be looking at is the hammer. Hammers are great instruments to use when we want to build something up, secure something down, or tear something apart. There are some unique things about this tool that make it ideal for improving our mental health. So grab your hammer and let's get going.

When you think of fixing something that's broken, a hammer is probably not the first tool that comes to mind. And when talking about broken people, a hammer may seem a little extreme. Hammers have a bad rap for causing pain and breaking stuff. But when used correctly, with practiced skill and expertise, hammers are actually one of the best tools for protecting things from getting broken and fixing them when they are.

I'd really love to have a super-smooth way to say, "Hey, folks. Here's a hammer, and I'm going to be using it as an analogy for journaling," but I don't. I'm just going to do a lot of comparing and, in the end, hope that you think I am an incredible genius like my dog thinks I am. So yeah, hammer = journal.

I suspect that upon hearing the word journal, you are already looking for your receipt and wondering if you can still get a full refund for this book. I get it. I do. A journal can be extremely awkward and even dangerous if not used properly. Most of the chapters in this section are devoted to winning you over and offering useful instruction on how to get it to work well for you with as little pain as possible.

Don't worry, I see you out there, too, Journaling Freaks. You with your "I love my journal" coffee mugs, lapel pins, and t-shirts. Ya'll are a crazy bunch, and I love you for it. You have already experienced the powerful tool that a journal can be. I've got some stuff in here for you, too. Stuff to keep you thinking. I'm confident your passion will be ignited by new thoughts and ideas, inspiring you toward new ways of journaling.

Me? I think journaling is super helpful, but unfortunately, I don't own the mug*. It's extremely valuable when I use it, but as with all things when dealing with a serious mental illness, it often gets forgotten or the task seems too overwhelming. If you're there like I have been, I've got some easy and exciting tips in here for you as well.

So whether you hate journaling or you love it, I want to challenge you to read through the following chapters slowly and consider many of its benefits. It's not a coincidence that it's the second tool we're looking at. When I first started writing this book, I knew—and had experienced—that journaling was a vitally important part of my mental health and well-being. I just couldn't really explain why. I can, now. I will, here. Let's dig in.

*An update about not having the coffee mug: one of my editors, upon reading that I did not have an "I love my journal" coffee mug decided to buy me one. So, three years after writing this section, I now have an "I love my journal" coffee mug, and I couldn't be happier.

JOURNALING'S REPUTATION

There are a lot of opinions out there about what journaling is and is not. Here's what I think: Journaling is taking what is in your head and/or heart—all those thoughts, ideas, creations, and imaginations that make you, well you—and brings them out and onto/into a tangible medium, typically for your eyes and ears only.

Sometimes I don't want to journal. And so, I don't. I don't have the time or can't think of anything to write. There are times that the mere thought of picking up a pen and chronicling how I feel will be the straw that breaks the camel's back. And to be honest, sometimes, I just plain forget to do it, or that it's really helpful for me.

And then there are times I can't get enough of it. The house is quiet. I'm wrapped in my favorite blanket, sitting in my favorite recliner, sipping on my favorite chocolate moo brew. There's a fan blowing nearby. And my teenage boys are singing sweet songs in beautiful harmony in the next room. Ok, that last part doesn't happen. But you get the idea. Sometimes I get in a mood. And that mood is very conducive to journaling.

What do you think about journaling? Do you think that most people who journal actually enjoy doing it? If you ask most people—professionals or otherwise—they will most likely tell you they think journaling is a good idea. But just because it's a good idea doesn't mean people actually like to do it. And it certainly doesn't mean that most people are doing it. It's like drinking water. We know it's is a good idea. We think about it when we want to get serious about self-improvement. Heck, we even want to want to do it. It's kind of a no brainer. Our bodies need water. And yet, do we get enough of it? I know I don't. Why not? For me, the answer is simple: Water is boring! When I drink something, I want instant gratification. I want taste. I want the buzz of sugar. I want excitement. There are times on a hot day or after an exhausting workout that I crave water, but usually, I want something else. Like water, journaling won't give you that exciting, instant rush. Its benefits, as great as they are, typically take time to reveal themselves. The changes are slow and incremental, but they are also deep and will have a huge, lasting impact on your quality of life.

Journaling may not be quite as important to us as water, but I'm convinced you will be impressed by just how transformative and beneficial spending even as little as two to five minutes a day doing it can be.

Maybe you've struggled with journaling? You are not alone. Lots of people avoid journaling, and I think one of the reason is social media. What do most people use Facebook for? It's a place to record experiences, express themselves, and share their opinions. People— myself included, spend a lot of time and emotional energy posting, replying, and liking posts that could be spent journaling. For me, it comes down to how I use my journal.

There are a few ways I use my journal: to remember the people and feelings of specific events, for self-expression/reflection, and for prayer. The basic and historic idea behind a journal is that it's something we use to store our secrets, not something that's meant to be shared with the general public. We don't ask people to take a look in our journal to see if they "like" an idea or opinion of ours. Nobody that I know of has a "reply" section underneath their journal entries. But just because it hasn't happened doesn't mean it's a bad idea. Journals are a great place to develop and critique your own ideas and opinions. It's a safe place to work out some of those things without fear of insult or injury.

What is so attractive about social media that has allowed it to run roughshod over journaling? Well, for starters, it meets the need for validation and instant gratification. Think about your most recent post expressing something you felt or thought. How long did it take to get a few likes or supportive comments? While writing this paragraph, I set a stopwatch next to my laptop and posted "I feel very relaxed." on Facebook.

Twenty-one seconds.

That's how long it took for someone to respond. That will never happen with a journal. Facebook, Twitter, and other social media platforms are extremely powerful—and sometimes even helpful tools, but once you learn the power of journaling, I think you will agree that we all should spend a little more time doing that than being on our devices.

*You*tilization

One thing that I've found that helps me journal, is having one that I like to look at. I have about twenty-five journals of various materials, shapes, sizes, and colors that span the last seventeen years of my life. It's exciting to find a good-looking journal that smells nice and feels great in my hands. Another thing that has made a big difference for me is my choice of writing instrument. I have had a lasting love affair with the Pilot G-2, (size: 0.07) for years, years, and years. It's a gel pen that won't freeze up in the winter and just feels wonderful to write with. You see that journaling is important, and now I want you to put your money where my mouth is. Find a journal at the local book store or online. One that screams "WRITE IN ME!" And then go get yourself a Pilot G-2.

THE POWER OF JOURNALING

On February 22nd, 2004, I had been married for about six years. There was no major event that happened on that day, only a simple prayer for courage and self-confidence in my marriage. I constantly write about my fears and perceived shortcomings because I always want to be moving forward. I always want to be doing better, whatever that means. A couple of days ago, on February 22nd, 2021, I was writing in my journal and thought, I wonder if I have a journal entry for this day in one of my older journals. I turned to my 2004 journal and saw that I had. I then began to remember the fear and doubt that used to consume me. I can't express how wonderful and encouraging it feels to see the growth that I have experienced in the last fifteen years. I have no doubt that journaling played a humongous role in my personal growth. This chapter is devoted to the two biggest reasons why journaling is such an amazing tool.

There's an article I read not too long ago that sealed the deal for me in regards to journaling. In *The Life-Changing Habit of Journaling* by Thomas Oppong, he says, "Journaling is not a commonplace habit, it is a **keystone habit**. Keystone habits affect how you work, eat, play, live, spend, and communicate. A minor change in one aspect of your life can trigger so many other positive changes." He continues to say, "Journaling is a practical and accessible way to stay connected to your inner self, your body, your dreams and your purpose in life." Charles Duhigg, author of *The Power of Habit* says, "[Keystone habits] encourage change by creating structures that help other habits to flourish."

But wait, there's more!

In the article *What are Keystone Habits?* written by Steve Scott, he reinforces that they "… lead to the development of multiple good habits. They start a **chain [reaction]** in your life that produces a number of positive outcomes." Ok. Stop everything. Do you see it? Your journal isn't just a tool, it's a superhero! I mean, minus the cape, utility belt, and spandex, this thing is crazy-powerful.

This is a really big deal. A chain reaction, according to the Merriam-Webster online dictionary, is "a number of events triggered by the same initial event." Are you getting this? When we journal, we begin to set in motion a series of events that take on a life of their own.

As I write this section, I'm camping with my oldest son. One of the better moments of our trip happened while we were throwing stuff into the lake. We started off small, finding pebbles and small branches to toss in. In no time, we began looking for the biggest objects we could carry. It was both relaxing and fascinating to watch the ripples expand from even the smallest object disturbing the surface of the water. My son would grab a stick, toss it out, and watch as the water danced away from the point of impact, traveling in all directions until ultimately fading away or reaching the shoreline. (Yeah, we're most definitely nerds like that.)

The final, barely noticeable ripples touching the shore can be directly linked through causation to the stick. They operate completely independent of the now floating chunk of wood.

They.

Did you catch that? Have you ever noticed that there's not just one ripple but many ripples that coexist in a pattern that seems uniform and organized? This is the beauty of a chain reaction! It's the change in something—in this case the water—caused by an initial action, something hitting the surface of the water.

How does this relate to journaling? Journaling is like that stick impacting the water. It takes initial effort and intention to get the stick in the air/to write in your journal. This sets in motion multiple elements of your life, acting in unison to create a pattern, beauty, and flow to life. When that stick leaves your hand/you write in your journal, a whole series of events are set in motion that are out of your control. I can't wait for you to get to the next few chapters and read some of the specific benefits journaling is capable of having in your life.

*You*tilization

I've introduced you to two fundamental and super-duper awesome aspects of journaling: Keystone Habits cause a Chain Reaction throughout your life. For this exercise, I'd like you to grab some sticky notes (or slips of paper) and some tape and make a list of three areas of your life you wish would improve (one per paper). Then, stick them on the next blank page. I want you to remember these as you continue reading.

Sticky Notes
Go Here!

BENEFITS OF JOURNALING

So ... there's no spandex or cape, but you're getting ready see how super-powerful a journal can be. Who's your favorite superhero? Mine's probably Superman. He can fly, has x-ray vision, laser vision, super breath, strength, and speed. If you could have a special power, what would it be? Would you like to fly? Run faster than a locomotive? Leap tall buildings in a single bound? Well ... unless you were born on a different planet and sent to earth in a rocket ship, you're probably out of luck. So, what ARE some of journaling's superpowers? What if I told you it can help you be a better friend? Parent? Spouse? You'd probably believe me. But what about better at sports? Wealthier? Smarter? Thinner? More employable? Healthier? If any of these things appeal to you, then a journal is just what you need.

You may be saying to yourself, "Self, this guy has got to be exaggerating!" My self would tell your self, "Hey, self of yours, this self is not exaggerating. This is legit." Check this out:

Benefits of Journaling: Journaling and Friendship

I'm not going to spend too much time here because the topic comes up later in the book, but let me at least say this: I love being intentional with my friends. I like to plan, to surprise them, and to remember things we've done together—the good times, that is. I think a journal is a stellar place to keep all this important stuff, don't you?

Benefits of Journaling: Journaling and Parenting

I spoke to a mom recently, my friend Jennifer, and asked her for her feelings about journaling. She's a missionary in Mongolia, a wife, and a mom of a pre-teen. There are a few things she brought up that really stood out to me about parenting. First, she mentioned that having a journal gives you a safe space to process your emotions and thoughts without offending or hurting anyone's feelings. Having a place to think about the words you are going to say to your child is a really good idea. She also mentioned that journaling helps her determine if the goals she is setting for herself and her daughter are healthy and reasonable. She can work through potential outcomes to see how things may play out in the future. Lastly, having a journal as a parent can be extremely encouraging. When you take the time to look through past journals and see the stories and struggles of your family, it can be a beacon of hope that reminds you that whatever you may be going through right now will probably be a distant memory someday. And if you made it through all that stuff in those past journals, you can certainly make it past this next obstacle.

Journaling and Our Bodies

Being able to have that outlet to express feelings in a safe place is a great tool for moms and dads. We can not only sort out problems and clear our heads, but scientific research also shows that journaling can actually make us healthier. I have my own theory about this, but first, let's take a look at some of these findings about journaling.

The University of Iowa reported that "... meta-analysis of the effects of written disclosure [journaling] found that writing about stressful or traumatic events is related to improvements in self-reported health, psychological well-being, physiological functioning, and general functioning. Moreover, the positive effects of written disclosure appear to be equivalent to or greater than effects produced by other psychosocial interventions (Ullrich & Lutgendorf, 2002)."

Say what? Real quick, let's define psychosocial. From Study.com, "... we see that 'psycho' refers to psychology—the study of human nature or the mind, its functions, and behavior—and 'social' refers to society—groups of people living together with shared laws and organizations. If we put these two ideas together, we can see that psychosocial refers to how humans interact with and relate to others around them. It focuses on relationships and how humans work in society (Psychosocial Intervention, 2017)."

Essentially, the University of Iowa report is saying that journaling may surpass social benefits to our physical health. And all the introverts in the room rejoice … quietly … and in private! I'm not telling you to hide in your closet with a journal and a package of Mint Oreos and chocolate milk and you'll never get sick. Everything in moderation. Humans were created for community. You and I need each other. This may seem a little crazy, that simply writing in a journal can do so much, but when we consider our physiology and how it works, then maybe it will make a little more sense.

Physiology refers to the function of the human body and its parts, all the way down to the molecular level—the smallest parts of what makes us 'us.' A house isn't just a collection of wood, bricks, wires, and plumbing. No, it's a combination of these materials *and* the action that organized them. Bricks don't lay themselves and then call it a house. They need builders. These builders in our bodies are neurological chemicals that operate and are instructed from our brains, which respond to our environment, thoughts, and emotions. The response to specific instructions (the doing), along with the appropriate materials (the chemicals), is what causes houses to be built—and, interestingly enough— bodies to heal and maintain health. When you take the time to journal, you are effectively giving your body instruction to function in a healthy way. From a spiritual perspective, this strikes me as absolutely true. 'Existence' couldn't exist merely by materials forming accidentally. There is thought, reason, and heart behind the existence of things. Sure, we are a bundle of chemicals and tissue. But that bundle doesn't just form itself. No, I believe it had an ultimate builder. But I digress.

Here are just a few physical benefits of journaling reported by the American Psychological Association (Murray, 2002):

- boosts immune functions with patients having HIV/AIDS, arthritis, and asthma

- lowers blood pressure

- improves the body's response to the Hepatitis B vaccine

- reduces deterioration for those with asthma and arthritis

- weight loss

The overall conclusion is that journaling is focused on emotional disclosure (writing about our feelings) and cognitive processing (writing about thoughts related to those feelings) and is therefore, really, REALLY good for our minds and bodies.

Journaling and Our Bodies: Weight Management

In 2013, CNN published an online article reporting on the effectiveness that journaling has on weight management. Supported by research that's documented in the *Journal of the Academy of Nutrition and Dietetics* as well as the *American Journal of Preventative Medicine*, the article says that keeping a journal about health-related habits has been proven to be an effective tool for managing weight. Charmaine Jackson, the subject of the article who went from 260 to 130 pounds, explained what journaling did for her. She said, "[It] really helped me get an idea of what my behaviors are, what my patterns are, and how I can make change[s] for myself for good (Caruso, 2013)." This reinforces the idea that journaling is a keystone habit. Writing in a journal won't melt the pounds away, but it will develop multiple life habits that lead to greater outcomes like weight loss.

No matter how you look at it, getting to and maintaining a healthy weight takes a lot of work. And Charmaine's story probably sounds like one of a thousand other stories you've heard before. Take this pill, drink this drink, eat this food, do this exercise, and the pounds will come off. So, what's so special about journaling? Journaling, in fact, is not a one off, super-secret, revolutionary method for weight management that is suddenly going to take the world by storm. Nope. Because it already has. You may not realize it, but the majority of effective healthy eating programs have been using some type of journaling method for generations. From Weight Watchers, that utilizes a food based points system, to the Mayo Clinic, which has a variety of journal type formats (Habit Tracker, Fitness Planner, and their own published *Mayo Clinic Diet Journal*), recording personal eating habits and setting goals has long been proven to be an effective route toward weight loss. This is confirmed by Doctor Jessica Barfield, of Loyola University Health Systems, who says in the same article that self-monitoring is a highly effective method of weight management. Counting calories is one aspect of that, she says, but other factors are when you eat (showing the gap between meals), how many fluids you are taking in—and the type, sleep habits, and how you are feeling emotionally. "[Charmaine] is just one great success story of the benefits of self-monitoring in the weight loss and management process (Caruso, 2013)." Use the Mental Health Scale when you journal, and you will have a quick and easy record of how you are feeling when you eat.

I think it's important to recognize that sometimes there are barriers to healthy living that go beyond merely managing your diet or exercising. Writing in a journal can be a great way to support and encourage yourself. It's also a great place to reflect on unhelpful/unhealthy social pressures to lose weight in the first place. Because journaling is a keystone habit, it's also an excellent tool that supports and reinforces **all** of the things that are necessary for healthy living and weight management.

Journaling and Our Bodies: Sports

In the *North American Journal of Psychology*, it was found that an athlete's mood affects his or her performance. In a study of collegiate tennis players, researchers divided the athletes up into one of two categories: mood monitors and mood labelers. Mood monitors are athletes who constantly keep tabs on their emotions. Mood labelers are people who notice emotions, label them, and then move on. It was observed that because of the high level of focus needed in the sport of tennis, mood monitors were at a disadvantage having "fewer cognitive resources to devote to the proper execution of the game (Scott, et al, 2003)." Researchers reported that this group benefited from emotive writing (aka, journaling about their moods and emotions) in the long run, experiencing measurable performance improvement. That makes sense, doesn't it? If a person is constantly focused on how they're feeling, it leaves them distracted from other activities. Therefore, having a place like a journal to express those emotions for later reflection, can drastically improve one's focus.

Managing and labeling moods are not the only ways to improve a person's athletic performance. Anyone can use a journal as a personal development tool by setting goals, tracking performance progress, and observing/reflecting on setbacks. These are all proven and effective ways to develop an athlete's personal abilities. Things like stamina, strength, agility, accuracy, and consistency are all things that are measurable and developable with the use of a personal journal. In addition, a journal is a great tool to help identify mental or emotional roadblocks to personal development, and then, also, a place to work through them toward a solution.

Life can be so complicated, can't it? We all wear so many different hats. You're a parent, chef, house cleaner, taxi service, psychologist, friend, teacher … the list goes on and on. And on top of all that, oh yeah, you need to try to keep yourself alive and healthy. That's all. Maybe a journal will help?

*You*tilization

First of all, I'd like you to go back to the Mental Health Scale. How are you feeling today? Tell a friend your Mental Health Number. If it's a rough day and you find yourself in the negatives, give yourself a break. You're doing the best you can!

Next, take a few minutes to take care of your body and mind today. Go for a walk and enjoy the fresh air and beauty of nature. Have you seen a dentist in a while? How about a physical with your primary care physician? Eye doctor? Light some candles and take a nice, long, hot bath or shower. You're a Broken Person on a journey toward wholeness.

Journaling and Your Money: Employment

This is what Monster.com has to say about journaling:

> "When was the last time you thought about how you can challenge yourself? Or took inventory of your accomplishments? Or even checked in with whether you're happy at work? Sometimes, you're so busy crossing tasks off a constantly growing to-do list that you're inadvertently neglecting your career performance and goals. You can reclaim that focus in as little as 15 minutes. How? By journaling at the end of every workday (Gross, 2021)."

Journaling is a fantastic skill that can be used to create or gain mental clarity, set goals, and to make plans for reaching those goals. Journaling was extremely helpful when I was seeking to advance my career at FedEx Express. I went through a two-year process of training, applying, interviewing, and being rejected for management positions all over the state. It was exhausting. Journaling was a great place for me to record my experiences, strategize for future interviews, and articulate my fears and frustrations with the process. It was also a place where I encouraged myself by recording goals, highlighting my strengths, and developing my unique leadership style. While journaling won't get you "the job", it can help you maintain your focus and motivation during the very long and frustrating process of finding that job.

Side note: I ended up getting a management job at FedEx after that two-year period at the location I most wanted, in my hometown of Grand Rapids, MI.

Journaling and Your Money: Financial

I'm a list person. That's what a big chunk of my journals contain, lists. Every week I write a grocery list in my journal. Quite often, my youngest son will tag along when I head out to the store. As we load up our cart, I write down the cost of each item, round it up to the nearest dollar, and keep track of how well we are doing versus the budgeted amount for grocery shopping. We've even made a game of it. If the total in my journal is significantly less than the actual total at the cash register, he gets a little cash for helping, and I buy us some kind of sweet reward.

Keeping a list like this has helped our family stay on budget. The game my son and I play is something that's evolved from just time shopping together, to discussions about how my wife and I use my journal and our budget to grocery shop. This is a super simple example of how my family has benefited both financially and relationally from journaling.

A 2018 *U.S. News and World Report* article (Hamm, 2018) said that there are four ways in which journaling can improve your financial situation. It can:

- help you think about how you spend your money,

- give you a platform for figuring how to accomplish specific financial goals, breaking them down into manageable tasks,

- be a tool to help you work through big financial decisions like finding a new job or saving for retirement,

- and offer you a place to process through uncertainty and worry.

Have you ever used one of those old-fashioned, fragile piggy banks? I've always wanted one just so I could use a hammer to break it open. Just like a hammer is an effective way to get money from a piggy bank, a journal is an effective way to break through barriers and reach financial success. It does so by giving you a handle on your budget while helping you smash through mental and emotional obstacles. Want to organize your goals and rally all of your scattered thoughts? Grab a pen and your journal! A person who spends their money wisely, with a plan, is far better off than a person who spends on a whim. Journaling is an absolutely fantastic tool to work on self-accountability and develop personal motivation.

One final thought about finances and journaling: Having a quiet place to reflect on and plan out all of the things that matter to you is super important. Thinking about money is one of those significant things. It's very reasonable, responsible, and necessary. But what if money is all you think about? I've always heard that the pursuit of riches is a never-ending journey. And if getting a lot of cash is your aim, you'll never have enough. Wiser people than I have said this. I've learned some pretty powerful lessons in life, much of which have come to me through personal reflections in my journal. I hope that journaling helps you to identify meaningful pursuits in life and enables you to stay focused on these things by removing stress caused by some of the more mundane things in life. I hope you will discover, as I have, that the important stuff that really matters in life, isn't something we can buy.

*You*tilization

What are some of your financial goals? Writing down your goals in a journal is an excellent way to begin accomplishing them. Strategize how you can achieve these goals, and reflect on setbacks and successes in relationship to your goals. Your journal is also a really good place to remind yourself of your priorities. How important is money in your life compared to say, your kids, your friends, or your health? And if your life isn't reflecting your priorities, journal about ideas that you can do something about it.

Journaling and Your Mind: Journaling to Know Yourself

One of the biggest challenges to writing a book is self-doubt. Add in mental illness, and you have a recipe for a casserole that will never be completely done. This chapter is weighing heavily on me right now, and I keep asking myself why. If I wait for it to be absolutely perfect, then this project will never get done. And I feel down to my core that it needs to get done asap. But this chapter wrestles with one of the most challenging and profound questions that I struggle to deal with (and most likely it's the same for you): "Who am I?"

It's tough! It really, really sucks when you have the free time and resources to do whatever it is you want to do but then can't figure out what that is. I remember asking myself in my late thirties what I wanted to be when I grew up. You'd think someone that old would already know the answer. But I had no idea. And to make matters worse, growing up in the church, I was taught that God had a specific plan and purpose for my life. The pressure of making sure I found the exact path God had for me only added to my anxiety.

A journal has been just the thing I've needed to sort through my issues. When I began discussing the journal a few chapters back, I introduced the hammer as an analogy. What is the main purpose of a hammer? To build, right? What does it build? Lots of stuff, but the first thing that comes to mind is houses. How does it build houses? Well, there's a pile of materials, some blueprints, and a bunch of experienced people who come together to do one thing... build. So, a hammer is a tool that takes boards and nails and brings them together into a stable, secure, and purposeful structure. Well, a journal is a tool that allows you to organize the pile of stuff that makes you you so that you can build confidence, and create support for personal stability, inner-security, and purpose! How?

First and foremost, a journal is such a helpful and safe place for us to determine the materials we have to work with. We figure this out by asking ourselves questions, and then answering as honestly as possible. They don't have to be—nor should they be—complicated questions. Remember, a hammer is just a simple tool used to bring boards and nails together. It's how they are brought together that's the hard part and requires a bit of experience. But we are getting there, so hold on!

Start by asking yourself about your likes and dislikes. What soda do you prefer? Did you enjoy your last meal? What things help you calm down? There are hundreds of questions you can ask yourself to identify your personal preferences. One of the complicating factors to figuring out who you are could be that you keep changing who you are, adjusting personal preferences to pacify or impress whoever you are currently hanging around with. Maybe your low self-esteem leads you to think there is something really wrong with you, while other people have it all together. At least, these are some of the common thoughts I have. I find myself not wanting to disagree with people I'm around for fear of losing that relationship. The result is, we keep the relationship... but lose ourselves.

Back to the hammer. There are lots of different structures that can be built with a hammer. Homes, gas stations, factories, and on and on. The differences all lie in the plans and materials, right? Most buildings share similar materials, but then there are things that are unique to the type and purpose of the specific structure being built at the time. Homes have a unique design that includes stairs, a fireplace, etc. A gas station has countertops, huge tanks, and complicated machinery. Factories are huge, with wide open spaces and large machines. Each building is unique and requires individualized plans and materials.

You are also unique! There are specific inner "materials" that make you you. When we are able to sort through all of the stuff we've allowed to pile up in our lives to find the materials that makes us us, then we can begin to see who we are and what we are capable of being.

So grab your journal, and ask yourself some easy questions. Start to identify your truest thoughts. You may discover that some of the things you have thought and believed your entire life are not actually your thoughts and beliefs. By being honest and allowing yourself space to process them, you may discover that you're wrong about some things. And if that doesn't scare you, then I don't know what will. But, guess what? Knowing what scares you is a super helpful thing to discover about yourself! When you find yourself bothered or afraid, be honest about it. Use that safe space in your journal to process through it.

As you identify all of your stuff (fears, beliefs, thoughts, etc.) and bring them together using a journal, you will begin to see purpose taking shape. Over time, you will feel the security of a house well built. And the satisfaction of having taken all these parts of you to truly figure out who you are.

A couple last points. One, a hammer isn't the only tool used to build, nor is it the best tool. Certain jobs require certain specialty tools. Regardless of the job, I can assure you that a hammer is always nearby—a ready tool to solve annoying problems. Drills and nail guns are some of the tools that have taken the place of hammers. In a similar way, there are specialty things/people in your life that are uniquely positioned to help you figure yourself out. These are your friends (which is something I can't wait for you to read about in the third part of this book), therapists, doctors, nutritionists, etc. All important. But there will always be the need for that simple hammer to keep around just in case.

And two, as you may have already determined, the question "Who am I?" is flawed. I feel like I am beating a dead horse here, but again the "Who am I?" issue is so important, and here's why. When someone asks you who you are, they don't actually want to know who you are. Complicated, right!? People really want to know what makes you unique, special, or different from everybody else. They are measuring your potential and making comparisons.

When someone looks at something and asks what it is, you tell them its given name. That big thing over there with a garage and a bunch of windows is called a house. When people ask who you are, the simple answer, in my case, is "I'm Joe." If the person asking you is interested or curious about you, they will need to know more. If someone is looking to buy a house, they will want to know what it looks like inside. They want to see what makes it unique. And when you're asked who you are, they want the same thing. They want to know what's inside. So make a list of what makes you you. Ask the simple questions. Just asking yourself questions and being unapologetically honest about your opinions in your journal is a great start. Then, dream about what you can do with all that stuff, and when you reach that point—as I know you will—where you have no clue what to do with all that weird and unique stuff that makes you you, that's when you can bring in the power tools and get more help. The friends, therapists, pastors, etc. Make a plan of who you will talk to, to find the answers you need when you don't understand how all of these pieces of you fit together.

Let yourself be you. The more often you do, the happier and more fulfilled you will be. And, even though happiness and personal fulfillment might not cure your mental illness, it sure does make living a bit easier and so much more enjoyable.

*You*tilization

This chapter covered a lot of ground! Take a second to evaluate how you are doing. What is your MHN today? Are you in a good spot, or do you need to make some forward motion?

Next? Make a list of some get-to-know-you questions. Think about a friend or a stranger. What questions would you ask to get better acquainted with them? Those are the things I also want you to ask yourself, with gut level honesty. You can answer them in your head or out loud, but I prefer a journal. Here are a few questions to get you started:

- What sport do you enjoy watching or playing?

- What music do you love?

- What music do you hate?

- What is one place you'd like to visit before you die?

Journaling and Your Emotions: The Kinesthetic Value of Journaling

While much of the information I've read about journaling speaks about the benefits that occur from sorting through mental or emotional issues, none of it has said anything about the kinesthetic value of the physical act of writing in a journal. I'm not talking about just putting thoughts down on paper. I'm referring to the actual scraping and gliding of the writing instrument on the surface of the paper.

Here's my two cents: I've been hospitalized for depression on two separate occasions. Each time I've been on one of these mini-emotional-getaways, I've found myself drawn to pencil and paper as a means of relaxation and distraction. I don't think this is a coincidence. There is certainly something to be said about getting away from technology and embracing a more hands-on, almost archaic, form of self-expression. Why did I do this, every time? Here's one idea I came up with: Have you ever run a vacuum to quiet a crying baby? Or taken them for a car ride just to get them to settle? Do you or someone you know use a fan, even in the dead of winter, to help you sleep at night? These are things that sooth us. It's not rocket science. It's white noise. It's the calming consistency of sound hitting our ears, distracting us from thoughts that would otherwise worry or consume us in restful, quiet times of our day or night.

What is sound? Sound is simply tiny vibrations hitting the eardrum. When I draw, the flow and grind of the pencil against the paper creates these tiny vibrations that help me calm down. I get distracted by the intensity of my attention and creativity when I focus on my drawing, lulled by the sweeping and soft wearing down of the graphite against the texture of the page. Just be careful not to overthink it. Don't do a lot of judging, and for goodness sakes, lower your personal expectations. It's not about how well you draw. This isn't a competition. It's self-expression which is best done when incorporated with self-directed kindness.

Journaling and Your Emotions:
The Emotional Benefits of Journaling

Here's the practical side of things: Let's say you're journaling at the beginning of the day because you're stuck in bed and can't think straight. Maybe you had a bad dream, had a bad experience the day before, or have a difficult situation to deal with that day. Journaling about it can help clear your mind, organize your thoughts, and make sense out of complicated and complex emotions. It may also provide clarity as you *you*tilize the logical part of your brain, while encouraging creative problem solving by freeing up the imaginative part of your mind. Remember the ripples from my camping trip? Those analogous ripples expand from the place that the stick (your journaling) hits the water. Writing stuff down is a great way to ease tension and reduce stress. And easing tension and reducing stress is a great way to enjoy your time with others and, more importantly, yourself. There can be a reduction of stress and increased relaxation by utilizing a writing instrument and paper and experiencing the calming sensations associated with this physical activity. We function and feel better when we are less stressed. Imagine what you'd be capable of accomplishing without it. Let me walk you through a recent event in which journaling played a key role in getting me moving in the right direction.

Journal Entry:

> *08-25-18*
>
> *Wow! Tough morning. Stuck in bed. What's bothering you? First of all, my body is really comfortable. I spent some time on Facebook wanting to see if people like me. My muscles are still sore from a workout two days ago.*
>
> *I'm dreading picking up the boys today. It's a long drive, and my car sucks. It's not fun to drive.*
>
> *What else are you feeling? I am feeling very sexually tempted to look at things I shouldn't. Thinking about things I shouldn't.*

What do you want to do today? Finish writing my chapter on journaling! I would like to finish reading Water Walker. I don't have time to do all of that and pick up the boys. I'm thinking about leaving super early just to get out there and chill.

I am actually feeling a little scared to get out of bed and face life. To leave my room and see all of my failures. Why does it have to be all about failures? Could you walk out of the room and possibly see all of the things you've done? Seriously?

Of course you'll notice things undone, but then look at the things you've accomplished.

But what's the purpose of it all? Why do we struggle? Why do we toil? For the act of love.

I feel like I'm not doing enough. Like I am missing it. There is always so much to do, to stress about.

It's been a privilege to lie in bed till 10 a.m. That's how I choose to look at it. Time to get up and make the day come alive. Time to do some amazing things!

This journal entry was that stick. I wrote it, threw it into the waters of life, and guess what happened? Ripples. Beautiful ripples. As mentioned in the journal entry, this was written at ten a.m. By ten-thirty, I forgot all about the struggle that had been keeping me in bed. This is how the day went for me: I was at the gym by ten-thirty, going through my workout routine. A couple of hiccups happened that morning: there was some confusion about when I was supposed to pick up my boys who were with their grandparents a few hours away, and then I was called by my mother-in-law to do something for her. I went home, took care of her, and then headed out to the pick-up spot, knowing that I would be a few hours early. And being early was just fine, because I really had no idea when I'd be meeting up to get my boy and I hate being late.

One of the big stressors of this trip was that my car sucked. It stalled at stoplights, and the brakes were not one-hundred percent reliable. (Don't try this at home, kids.) I brought my journal, an audio book, and my laptop to work on this book while I waited. I ended up getting to the pick-up spot about four hours before my boys arrived. It was extremely relaxing. I found a seat at a picnic table outside of a McDonald's and worked on my book. It was a beautiful day!

Then, something unexpected happened. A guy sat down at the adjacent picnic table, facing me. There were four other tables, which made his choice of seating a little awkward for me. Then he whipped out several ketchup packets and a plastic bowl of ice cream … from his backpack? When he started squeezing the ketchup onto the ice cream, I was fascinated (and slightly disturbed). Odd things like that really impress me, and so I asked him, "Did you really just put ketchup on your ice cream?" "Nope," he said. "It's potato salad." Side thought: is that any better? But, I digress. And just like that, it was like I pulled the pin on a conversational grenade. He exploded into a dialogue about his life. It was a pleasant conversation. But, being the introvert that I am and having a predisposition to selfishness, I just wanted to sit quietly and work on my book. Eventually, the concussive force of that grenade wore off and his social needs were satisfied … until my wife called. We spoke for a few minutes, all the while I could tell my new friend was listening intently. I told her about the ice cream/potato salad eating, ketchup coating guy at the table next to me, knowing he would get a kick out of hearing me talk about him. After hanging up, the guy asked me about the stickers on the back of my computer—I have a wide assortment there to create curiosity and draw attention to myself. You may think this sounds like self-sabotage for an introvert. You're probably right. Dang it!

At one point in the conversation, the subject of my mental illness came up. He began to share with me that he was homeless and looking for place to live, which lead to me telling him about my church and my beliefs in God. I gave him a tip on a shelter in Grand Rapids, along with a phone number. He was extremely thankful. It was an abnormal encounter, but pleasant, and I am glad it happened.

Let's go through the timeline of events and take a look at each ripple that day:

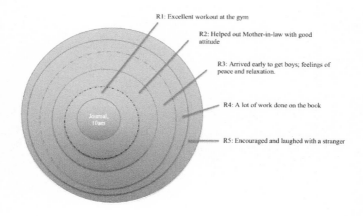

R1: Excellent workout at the gym

R2: Helped out Mother-in-law with good attitude

R3: Arrived early to get boys; feelings of peace and relaxation.

R4: A lot of work done on the book

R5: Encouraged and laughed with a stranger

Journal, 10am

My initial action, journaling, was the stick being tossed in the water. A ripple was formed, and I was at the gym. The ripples moved. I was physically and emotionally able to help my mother-in-law. From there I went to pick up my boys, arriving hours early at my destination to work on a book that may be helpful to thousands of people. The ripples continued. Next, I met a stranger from a completely different city, and we mutually encouraged each other through open conversation. This led to a pleasant conversation with the love of my life, that resulted in a further—more vulnerable—discussion with this gentleman about faith, finances, and life.

What if I didn't journal? Take a look at how I see that day playing out differently.

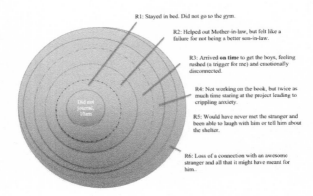

R1: Stayed in bed. Did not go to the gym.

R2: Helped out Mother-in-law, but felt like a failure for not being a better son-in-law.

R3: Arrived **on time** to get the boys, feeling rushed (a trigger for me) and emotionally disconnected.

R4: Not working on the book, but twice as much time staring at the project leading to crippling anxiety.

R5: Would have never met the stranger and been able to laugh with him or tell him about the shelter.

R6: Loss of a connection with an awesome stranger and all that it might have meant for him..

Did not journal, 10am

Great ideas and solutions to problems have a tendency to come when we are most relaxed and free from stress. That's one of the many ways journaling works. In a chapter in his fantastic book *The Happiness Equation* (please order this right now!) Neil Pasricha introduces us to the three B's of problem solving: Bed, Bathtub, and Bus. He suggests that some of the greatest discoveries ever made didn't happen in moments of stress and deep, intentional study, but in times of relaxation and leisure. He quotes Keith Sawyer, author of *Explaining Creativity*, saying,

"When we take time off from working on a problem, we change what we're doing and our context, and that activates different areas of our brains. If the answer wasn't in the part of the brain we were using, it might be in another. If we're lucky, in the next we may hear or see something that relates, distantly, to the problem we had temporarily put aside."

Consider these examples that Pasricha uses in his book: Where did Newton discover gravity? Sitting under an apple tree. How did Niels Bohr discover the structure of an atom? He was led by strange images in his dreams. Where did Archimedes discover that the volume of irregular objects could be measured by water displacement? He was stepping into a bath and noticed the water spill out of the tub.

I'm in a beautiful place to be writing a chapter about journaling, nearing the third day of this four-day wilderness father-son camping trip. If I could choose the perfect place to do some journaling, it would be right where I am at this moment: sitting in my green canvas camping chair on the moss-covered shoreline of a small lake, surrounded by lively, towering trees in the Manistee Huron National Forest. If you haven't had the chance to rest your bare feet on fresh, live moss, you don't know what you're missing. I've got my hiking boots off and am letting my feet relax, breathe, and stretch on the soft, cool texture of the ground. It is quite the relief after a day of sawing, cooking, sweating, and moving around. Having a journal that you enjoy writing in, a pen you like using, and a special place to write, is a fantastic formula for good journaling. "But I hate journaling," you say? Ah! We are about to get to that!

*You*tilization

Remember those sticky notes? Take a second to go back and look at them. They were the three things you'd like to see changed or affected in your life. Write them below, next to the three ripples, in order of importance. The most important change closest to the journal picture, and so on.

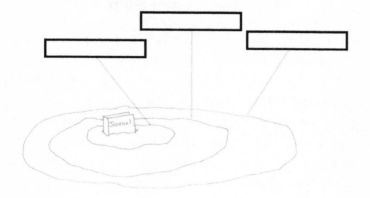

Original artwork by Joe Reid

JOURNALING OPTIONS FOR JOURNAL HATERS

Technology Based Solutions

As a young father, I did my best to adapt to the new experiences I faced with my precious daughter, Olivia. One of the hardest things I had to learn to deal with was bodily fluids (and solids). The diaper thing was still fairly new to me. The daddy thing was new. Heck, my marriage was relatively new. So, when I ran out of diapers one day while my wife was out with our only car, I got creative! With a pair of my tightie-whities and a few strategically-placed staples, I had found my solution. Voilá, problem solved. Insta-diaper!

So, ok, my diaper solution was less than perfect. But it sure did make me feel good to have adapted. That's what I want you to consider doing with this next chapter: adapt. Don't like journaling? Adapt. Give other alternatives a shot. Love journaling? Maybe you'll love it even more when you consider other options!

You are different. It doesn't matter how long you've known someone, if they're related, or your spouse, there's no one just like you. You are unique. My wife and I are a perfect example. We've been together for over twenty-five years, get along and work together as a team pretty well; but we are far from being "alike." She likes coffee; I like hot chocolate. She's a Starbucks fan; I prefer Biggby. She likes a glass of wine; I crave ice cold southern tea. She puts her children in diapers; I … adapt. We are all very different people.

Another difference between us is our preference for journaling. I prefer it, while she prefers to do anything but. This got me thinking. How can someone who hates journaling receive the benefits of it without actually doing it? "Impossible," you say? (If you didn't say it, would you say it right now? It will make me feel better.) That's what this section is about; Options! Even if you love journaling, here are some other ways you may not have considered (and the four I will be highlighting):

- video journaling

- audio journaling

- journaling apps

- e-journaling

If you own a smart phone or laptop, these options are a cinch. If you've given up on journaling, I hope you'll consider one of these technology-based avenues of self-reflection and exploration.

Journaling Options for Journal Haters: Video Journaling

Grab a cup of coffee. Find a quiet spot. Place your cellphone facing you on a table or in your lap. Take a deep breath. Click record and start talking. That's all there is to it. One of my friends, Caleb, prefers video journaling. He likes it because he is intrigued by the personal change he sees in himself as he grows older. When you write in a journal, you're able to read about how you handle life's problems and deal with stress differently as you mature. In a video journal, you get all of that plus the added bonus of literally seeing yourself handle life's problems, deal with stress, and how it affects you right before your eyes. How cool is that?

If you are visiting a new or unique place, create a video journal while giving a walking tutorial/tour. I did this while walking the streets of a small town in central Africa (Blantyre, Malawi). There was so much activity. So many new sounds. So many different kinds of people. Creating that video was a very emotional experience for me. I was able to record things I found interesting and, at the same time, capture my emotions in the moment. Priceless!

Human beings communicate on so many more levels than words. In 1971, Albert Mehrabian wrote the book *Silent Messages* in which he explained the results of an experiment that has led to some confusion over the years. There is a common statistic floating around, accredited to this one study, that humans communicate seven percent of their message with words and ninety-three percent with non-verbal communication. This is a ridiculous claim—not because Albert was wrong, but because the results of his study have morphed into saying something the researcher never intended to say. The study asked participants to listen to the single word, "maybe," and then try to determine whether the word that was said expressed a liking, disliking, or neutral emotion. Then they were given pictures expressing the same feelings at a separate time. The participants guessed the actual feeling correctly fifty percent more often with the pictures than with the way the word was said. This doesn't prove that it's more important how you say something than what you said, it just proves that a single word said may be more difficult to interpret than the facial expressions conveying that emotion. So I won't be using that statistic, but we cannot disregard that we do communicate a lot with facial expressions and tone of voice, things that are absent in a paper and pen journal, but are added benefits of a video journal. Learning to manage facial expressions during important conversations can be critical to getting your intended point across.

Journaling Options for Journal Haters: Audio Journaling

I've done audio journaling a couple of times. One of the things I like most about this option, is its convenience. Just like with video journaling, all you need is your mobile device. I tend to think audio journaling is more convenient than video journaling though, for a few reasons. With audio journaling, you don't have to worry about lighting. Video journaling requires at least some light, or what's the point? If you're in a poorly lit room, or just riding your bike down the street, you can audio record your thoughts without concern for what is seen. Additionally, audio journals can be made in the presence of considerably more background noise than a video journal because the mic to source (your mouth) distance required is much smaller. With an audio journal, you still get the added benefit of observing some change, but obviously it's limited to only the things you can hear.

If you are in a crowded area and need to process your emotions or remember an important thought, this would be a great opportunity to create an audio recording! What's fun about this? Just pretend to be having a conversation on the phone while venting and/or recording your ideas; it's sneaky, but who doesn't love a little subterfuge?

Video and audio journaling are also great ways to practice and improve speech. This was another one of the benefits my friend Caleb told me about. He uses the video platform to practice his speaking and diction. It is also good practice when preparing for interviews and tough conversations.

Journaling Options for Journal Haters: Journaling Apps

Another way technology has made journaling easier is with journaling apps. There are dozens, maybe even hundreds, out there for your phone or tablet, but I'm going to take a second to focus on just one: Daylio.

Daylio, available in the App Store and on Google Play, allows you to record your mood during specific activities throughout the day. It literally takes seconds to use. It also provides space with each entry to make notes to describe your emotions and experiences in more detail. It's a super convenient tool. One additional benefit is that you can set up multiple alerts to remind you to use it regularly. This option is available after you purchase the premium app (currently $23.99 a year).

When you check out the Daylio app, you'll see that you can select several activities and moods multiple times a day. You can also add activities that aren't on the provided list. It tracks your moods based on activities and will open your eyes to see how your mood can change based on what you're doing or where you are. There are also great graphs and charts to help you visualize trends as well. You receive "rewards" when you post consistently, and you can also set up daily reminders to record how you are doing at certain times. It's a mostly free, simple tool with a lot of fun options.

Journaling Options for Journal Haters: E-journaling

The last technology-based method I want you to know about is the electronic journal, or e-journal for short. This type of journaling resembles the traditional paper and pen version, but it's done in a Word document or some other word processing format. The benefits are similar, but not exactly the same. First, most people can type faster than they write. So, getting your thoughts down as they come is easier. Second, you can file and recall specific information much quicker than with a traditional journal. A computer allows you to search its memory for a specific phrase. In addition, you can easily create multiple copies of the document and file them in different folders. Another option that's available when you e-journal is the ability to insert media: music, videos, and photos. I love this idea because there are significant pictures or songs that connect to life events. Do you remember that old saying, "A picture is worth a thousand words?" Yet another excellent reason to use this method. There are a ton of great things you can do when you're using technology! A journal entry could literally just be a picture.

One last note about technologically based journaling options. It's probably going to be awkward to start off. But like most things, give it time. The benefits of the process are just too huge to ignore!

Journaling for Journal Haters: Paper and Pen Alternatives

These are types of paper and pen methods and journals that I've used with varying degrees of success. They are free-writing, gratitude, nature, goal setting, prompting, micro-journaling, and prayer journals.

Paper and Pen Alternatives: Free-Writing

One format of journaling I often use is free-writing. It is literally just writing what you think when you think it. That's it. Think it. Write it. No matter how ridiculous. Don't judge yourself. No one else is going to judge you because they're not going to see it. It doesn't have to be legible, have punctuation, or proper spelling. This method is helpful to me because I am less likely to judge what or how I write. Don't forget, your journal is a safe place for you to be who you are without fear of judgment or ridicule. Free-writing has been such a helpful way for me to journal because I'm less focused on form and literary rules, and more focused on what is going on inside of me.

Paper and Pen Alternatives: Gratitude

Gratitude journaling is writing down what you are thankful for. There are a ton of great websites and books out there to guide you through this. Here are a couple of my favorites:

Neil Pasricha, author of *Happiness Equation*, also has the blog *1000 Awesome Things* (1000awesomethings.com). In his blog, he has a list (as the name suggests) of 1,000 awesome things. He's got things on there I hadn't previously considered being thankful for. But when I thought about how awesome they are, I began to pay a little more attention to other things I could be thankful for. For example: the gas arrow on your dashboard telling you which side your gas tank is on; being the first table to be called up to the buffet at a wedding reception; and the smell of bread. I like to stick my nose into the soft insides of a fresh loaf of bread and take a deep breath. I absolutely love that smell!

One Thousand Gifts: A Dare to Live Fully Right Where You Are by Ann Voskamp, encourages the reader to find joy in the little things of life, even the really tough stuff. You could probably check it out of the library, but you'll want to highlight the heck out of it; so just buy it. Here are a couple quotes from it that really caught my attention:

"I want to see beauty. In the ugly, in the sink, in the suffering, in the daily, in all the days before I die, the moments before I sleep."

"...the secret to joy is to keep seeking God where we doubt He is."

Ann encourages her readers to pay attention to all the wonderful gifts that exist around us. To look at the things we value, appreciate, and admire, and to make a list of these things as gifts to be grateful for. Here are some of mine: right angles, the color Canary Yellow, and the reflection of trees on a glassy lake.

Paper and Pen Alternatives: Goal-Setting

If you want to make significant changes in your life, then a goal-setting journal is for you. This type of journal will help you set and track personal goals. It's one of my favorite ways to journal! There are three basic steps I recommend for creating a goal-setting journal entry. One, decide what you want to do. Two, decide when you want it done by. And three, create a schedule/action plan to get it done. There are a ton of free websites and resources to help you get started:

1. StikK.com: This website gives you a wonderful platform to set goals.

You can set up referees who help you achieve your goal by monitoring your progress. One of the really great options is that you can set up financial incentives to accomplish your goals. You can designate a certain dollar amount to be donated to a charity of your choice if you do not follow through on the thing that you want to achieve. The website refers to this as "utilizing the psychological power of loss aversion and accountability to drive behavior change."

2. Goalscape.com: This website uses unique visual aids to help you reach your goal and makes it easy to adjust priorities.

3. Coach.me: This is an app that has both free and paid options. It is simple to use and with the paid option, you can get personalized direction from a coach.

Using these digital resources in tandem with your journaling will rock your world. Also, check with your local librarian for other books and resources to help you figure this stuff out. Libraries are such an awesome, oft forgotten, resource. And ... they're free!

Paper and Pen Alternatives: Prompting

If journaling is difficult for you because you can't think of what to write, one successful and fun option myself and a few other friends have used is a prompting journal. These journals ask questions or give prompts to get you thinking. You can choose to follow the prompt or do your own thing. The main thing is that the help is there if you need it.

Here are four different prompting journals I've used:

1. *A Father's Legacy* (ISBN: 9780849952753);

A Mother's Legacy (ISBN: 9781404113336). Publisher: Thomas Nelson

These are prompting journals that are meant to be passed on to your children. They ask questions about your history, dreams, hopes, values, and life experiences.

Here a few examples:

- "Share a memory about the way you proposed to Mom."

- "Describe your childhood home. What was your favorite room?"

- "Describe your grandparents. What did you enjoy most about them?"

2. *Jesus Freak Journal* (ISBN: 1577782097), Albury Publishing: This journal uses

Thought Starters as a means to get you writing. It was created to be paired with the book *Jesus Freak*, which is a history of martyrdom of Christ followers. Here's a few of the Thought Starters:

- "What is my passion today? What is the Lord speaking to my heart?"

- "These are the areas of my life in which God is training me right now; this is how I have grown."

- "If it were illegal to be a Christian, what evidence would there be to convict me?"

3. *Fitlosophy, Fitspiration Journal* (Goal Getter Journal, no ISBN available). This

journal has a lot going on. It is perfect for both the seasoned "journaler" or for someone just starting out!

There are eight sections to each day's entry:

- Three things I'm grateful for

- Goals for personal fitness

- What I like about me

- Rate your day: Move (how was your workout), Nourish (What did you eat and how was your energy level), Reflect (What was your mood today).

- Fit Tip: A tip about healthy living

- A space for open journaling

- A motivational quote

- This inspires me

This journal is fantastic for veteran journal writers like myself because it is very detailed and structured. At the same time, it can benefit the newbie "journaler" by inspiring thought and providing prompts.

4. *The Purpose-Driven Life Journal* (ISBN: 0310805554). This journal gets its ideas and questions from, and was created to be used with, the best-selling book by Pastor Rick Warren, *The Purpose Driven Life*. Every day has new questions or thoughts that seek to inspire deeper perspectives and self-reflection. Here are a few examples:

- "Who do I need to restore a broken relationship with today?"

- "What problem in my life has caused the greatest growth in me?"

- "What's holding me back from accepting God's call to serve him?"

Paper and Pen Alternatives: Micro-Journaling

Micro-journaling is just as simple as it sounds. One of the biggest annoyances I have with journaling is the idea that I have to write a lot. I'll touch a bit more on this in the rules of journaling chapter. Micro-journaling is just writing about your day in a few words or sentences to get your feeling or main point across.

Paper and Pen Alternatives: Prayer

Another common format for me is prayer journaling. I often use my journal for intimate conversations between me and God. This has really helped my relationship with him. It's not easy for me to pray the traditional way—hands folded, eyes closed. I get bored and distracted far too easily. Writing down my prayers has increased how often I pray and how focused I am while doing it. There are a couple simple things I do to make prayer journaling work for me. The first and most obvious thing is to write out the prayer. There are many great guides that provide instruction on how to pray. Here are a couple of acronyms that may help lead to a more meaningful prayer time for you. The most common one I've found is ACTS.

- A- ADORATION; tell God you appreciate him

- C- CONFESSION; tell him where you've fallen short

- T- THANKSGIVING; thank God for stuff

- S- SUPPLICATION; ask God for stuff

ACTS is widely used, but it's kind of confusing to me. I've been a Christian for over thirty-seven years and still get messed up with words like "adoration" and "supplication." Who talks like that anymore? One less widely known acronym—because I just made it up—is FART.

- F- FIND; find a place to hide, then shut the door

- A- ASK; ask God to do something

- R- REMEMBER; remember who God is

- T- THANK HIM; thank him because all the good stuff is from him

When you're not sure how you should pray, just remember to FART. In fact, try FARTing without ceasing (1 Thessalonians 5:17). Your family will thank you for it.

Some of you may ask if FARTing is really an appropriate way to talk to God. I'll admit, it sounds a bit juvenile. At the same time, it's easy to remember because it's funny. And if a silly, somewhat juvenile, acronym is what it takes to remind me how to have a meaningful conversation with God, then I ask, "Why not?"

After I've finished writing my prayers, sometimes I'll go back through and read them aloud. There's something significant about this second part that makes it seem all the more sincere and meaningful. When I write the prayer initially, it seems to be more about what is in my head. When I go back and read through the prayer, it feels like it's more about what's in my heart.

There is one unique bonus of prayer journaling that I think is pretty cool. When you write down your prayers for people you care about, leave a line between the prayers for different people. Sometimes I copy these pages, cut out the prayers I've prayed for specific people, and then given them to that person as a gift. It's just something I do at the end of the year to remind them they're loved.

Paper and Pen Alternatives: Nature

A nature journal is "like a personal journal or diary … to record your observations and reflect on them, but unlike a diary, a nature journal is used specifically to record your observations of, and thoughts on, nature. Take up nature journaling and you can end up learning more about nature *and* about yourself (How to make a nature journal, 2020)."

I'm gonna be honest with you for a second (I've heard it's a good policy, after all). This type of journaling initially sounded awful to me! Sitting around a lake, looking at trees, and writing stuff down sounds more like a punishment than a personal benefit. But as I sit here on the edge of a lake while I camp with my son, I can't help but be silenced, overwhelmed, and grateful for the sheer beauty and majesty of this place. And so, while I'm here in the midst of it all, I can definitely understand how this nature journaling thing could catch on!

Here are a few tips to get started:

- Pick a journal that is durable and suits what you plan to use it for. You can draw, color, or paint on the pages, which is why you want to plan ahead when picking the type of journal that you buy.

- Journal while you are there, observing nature.

- Plan ahead so you can bring the right equipment.

- Plan your time.

- Observe. It's less about recording and drawing and more about observing.

- Begin each journal entry with your location and the time of day.

- Take pictures if you're not into drawing.

- Use the experience to learn new things about nature.

*You*tilization

Did that feel like a lot? I hope so. I hope you realize, whether you enjoy journaling or not, that there are a lot of options! So here's what I want you to do: Go back through the chapter and circle one of the journaling options you'd like to try. And then ... wait for it .... I want you to try it, for a week. And make it awful. Actually try to do it as imperfectly as possible. The key is to just do it!

THIS IS HOW WE DO IT

The last few years, I've developed a system that works very well for me. There are a few very specific reasons for this, which I will get to in a moment. Because I am a list, goal-oriented individual, my journal is naturally going to follow suit.

A few years ago, I made an exhaustive (and exhausting) list of everything I could think of in my life that mattered to me. Then I added all of the things I thought **should** matter to me. It was quite a long list. I then organized them into a few basic categories. The four I came up with were: God, Health, Family, Joe (Myself)

I put the four priorities at the top of the page like this:

God   **Health**   **Family**   **Joe**

The next thing I did was list all the tasks I needed and wanted to accomplish that day. Because each category was extremely important to me, I made sure to have at least one item under each. It usually looked something like this:

God	**Health**	**Family**	**Joe**
Bible Time	Medication	Read to wife	Read
Prayer	Gym	Read to my son	Friend-time
	Water x4	Helpful chore	

This became such a helpful part of journaling that I still use it today. After I make my lists, I do what I consider to be "normal journaling". I write about what happened or how I was feeling that day. Oftentimes I write about something I did wrong and how I can do it better. How's my marriage? How are my kids? What am I working on to improve my life? I'm always mixing it up. I get it, it's hard to write down this stuff. And guess what makes it harder? Unrealistic or burdensome expectations. The most consistent thing I do in my journal, as I mentioned earlier in the book, is make my list and pray. This is very helpful for my mental health, and is, by far, also the most helpful and healthy thing I do for my spiritual growth.

*You*tilization

One of the reasons I created the "God, Health, Family, and Joe" list is because it can be easy for me to feel overwhelmed in my day and not know what to do with myself. Setting small goals in each category gives me a starting point to get myself moving forward. It acts like a prompting journal... a template for my journaling life. Here's what I'd like you to do: Create your own prompting journal/ template. When you feel overwhelmed with life and don't know what to do, a journal, just like a close friend, is a great place to turn. Creating a template like mine will take the guess-work out of the process. You will use the logical side of your brain, because the emotional side is all discombobulated. Think about your life priorities and then categorize them. My friend Mike has six categories he focuses on every day. It doesn't matter how many you have as long as they are important and work for you.

Rules for Journaling

The next three pages are devoted to the sometimes-overwhelming rules that should be applied in any journaling situation regardless of the medium.

BROKEN LIKE ME

JOSEPH REID

As you can see, I don't think you need to worry about breaking any of the rules.

*You*tilization

What are some of your own self-imposed rules about journaling? I have preferences, but I am constantly changing how I do things because I get bored so easily. Grab your journal and write down some of the preconceived ideas that you've had about journaling.

FINAL THOUGHTS AND
A BRIEF WORD OF CAUTION

I. had. the. best. grandmother. ever. Her name was Lois Evelyn Chalcraft, but my kids called her Grandma Roses. She was thoughtful, patient, encouraging, and openly imperfect. When our kids were younger, we used to drive across the state to visit with family and would stay in the front bedroom of her two bedroom, single-wide trailer. Every morning, without fail, Grandma would grab the kids when they woke up, before they got too noisy and woke my wife or I. She'd make breakfast, usually French toast. I can still smell the butter cooking in the pan and the sweet syrup even now. She'd have my girls doing crafts at the kitchen table—usually those paper chains made with construction paper. It was always so important to her that I get enough rest. She had a lot of, what I sometimes think of as, old-fashioned rules. Don't slouch. Don't wear your hat at the table. And then there is the one about the face. I'll get to that in a minute.

Journaling is a lot like swinging a hammer. If there's a problem I'm trying to solve or I'm stuck in an emotional storm, I use my journal to help anchor me. It calms me down and gives me a safe place to process my thoughts. It's a wonderful tool, but just like with a hammer, you need to wield it with care. It's never a good idea to haphazardly swing a hammer around. If you're careless with it, someone's gonna get seriously hurt or stuff is gonna get smashed. It's also never a good idea to carelessly swing words around. Even when you journal, balance and moderation is key.

Here's the danger. When you're hammering a nail, you focus on that nail, aim, and swing. You don't close your eyes and hope you hit your mark. When you journal, it is equally important to think about what you are thinking about. To take aim with your thoughts and swing them toward a purposeful goal. With a hammer, you want to drive a nail into a stable place. With your journal, you want to drive your thoughts and emotions into a stable place as well. Take some advice from my Grandma. She didn't like seeing a sour face on her grandkids. She'd frequently tell us, "If you keep making that face, it's going to get stuck that way." I think the same goes for journaling. If your journaling is filled with negativity and constant complaining, without any thoughtful reflection or self-encouragement, your life is going to get stuck that way. It's ok to put the negative stuff in there but portion it out with a bit of self-reflection, celebration, problem-solving, hopes, and dreams for the future.

A journal is one of the most amazing and helpful items in your mental health tool box. It's an effective Keystone Habit that countless successful people have used throughout history to improve and manage life and emotional health. Why? Because it is so simple *and* it works! The key is to find the way it will work for you, and then use it. That's what *You*tilization is all about!

*You*tilization

There are a lot of tools in life that are meant to be helpful and good, but if used incorrectly, or without experience, can lead to some very unfavorable outcomes. Grab your journal and write down three tools that you use or are familiar with. Then, I want you to brainstorm how those tools are used for good, and right below that, how, when misused, they can cause pain or harm. Don't work with any tools? What about the telephone, the garbage disposal, or your car?

Wanna go even deeper?

Do you think that what you think a lot about affects how you perceive the world around you? Answer these questions in your journal: How can a journal be used to change how you think? And how can how you think change the world?

The
Third Tool

NAILING IT

It's time for us to go back to our trusty, rusty, red toolbox and see what other tools there are for us to use. Ok, so the measuring tape is on top. There's the hammer. Let's set those aside and see what else we've got. At the very bottom, we find a small, flimsy cardboard box. It rattles when we pick it up and sounds like metal. Nails probably? Be careful. Let's set it somewhere so we can check out what's inside.

Ok, crack it open. Just as we thought: nails. Nailed it! Go figure, there's got to be a dozen different kinds. They lay haphazardly arranged at the bottom of the box, are a dull, metallic gray color, have a little bit of gathered sawdust from past projects, and, oh look, a dead housefly wedged in a corner flap.

Pick a nail up. What do you think about its weight? Pretty light, right?

Try to bend it. Nope, not gonna happen. It is just a puny nail, but you still can't bend it. Hold the nail in your left hand between your thumb and index finger, pointy side up, as your right index finger examines the sharpened end. Flip it over, inspect the flattened head meant to make your aim true. There it is, flat and cold; only slightly bigger than the nail itself. I'm going to use this third tool to talk about friendship.

What is a nail? It's such a common thing people use. We see them everywhere, but do we truly understand what they are? Do we really appreciate what they do? What are friendships? They're such a common thing people have. We see them everywhere, but do we truly understand what they are? Do we really appreciate what they do? The dictionary defines a nail as, "a metal spike meant to hold things together," and friendship as, "a bond of affection or esteem meant to hold two or more people together."

When you see a nail, what do you think? Depends on where you see it, right? When we see nails holding the frame of a house together, we see them as helpful and necessary. If we find a nail on a counter, we might see it as clutter, then put it away where it belongs. If there's one on our living room floor, we'd pick it up because we wouldn't want someone to step on it and get hurt. If we've got one in our tire, well, that leads to a flurry of other emotions.

When you look at your friends, what do you think? Do you see them as helpful and necessary, helping you to keep it together? Do they get in the way, trying to monopolize your time? Are they supportive? Are they where you need them, when you need them? Do you have friends who cause hurt more than help? Are there friends in your life that stick into your emotional tires, puncturing your joy, making moving forward in life extremely difficult? After you've taken a second to answer these questions, why not give some thought to the type of friend *you* are.

This part of the book is all about friendship. Friendship is one of the most important tools we can have to help us work toward mental wellness. It helps us deal with the daily, sometimes minute to minute, challenges of having a mental illness. Healthy friendships can be more important than medication, exercise, and rest. Why? Because friends will help us remember and encourage us to do these things. Good friends will be honest with us if something we're doing doesn't seem to be working. These people will point out our strengths, celebrate our victories, and walk alongside us in our trials. They will confront us when we make bad decisions. Yes, friendship is unquestionably an important tool.

Hardware stores are filled with all sorts of tools and supplies. When you find the nail aisle, you may be surprised to see just how many types there are; different kinds, made from different materials, because different jobs require different specifications. When you consider spending time with someone, you're really opening up a door to your heart. I've found that having a variety of friends is invaluable and necessary. You've got different friends, made from different experiences, because different seasons of life sometimes bring different people.

A common nail weighs very little. You can carry dozens of them without feeling weighed down. Of course, if you carry them incorrectly, you're gonna know they're there. I remember carrying some in the pocket of my jeans one time. They jabbed the side of my leg whenever I moved. Annoying as heck. Friendships, as a rule, shouldn't feel like that. Friends shouldn't be a burden. If you feel hurt by a friend, first take a good look at how you're treating them. Just like pants pockets are not the ideal place to carry nails, mishandling friendships can lead to unnecessary pain, not because of what they did, but because of something you did. There will be times when a friend hurts you, because you can't escape the fact that friends are people; and people can be unpredictable, emotional, and selfish. Why? Because everybody, our friends included, has problems. Which leads to a major component of friendship: we carry each other's burdens.

Nails are deceptively strong. They have to be, right? What about our friends? Do friends have to be strong? Absolutely. There's a problem though: most of us have trouble recognizing those strengths. You've undoubtedly heard that beauty is in the eye of the beholder. I am convinced that strength is too. You don't have to be ripped with muscles to be considered "strong." The kind of strength we need from our friends, that strength that will get us through the day, goes much deeper than that. I'm talking about simple compassion, faithfulness, love, loyalty, and kindness. My strength is empathy, the ability to feel and relate to what others feel;

the ability to get it. That's what friends need, strength that goes far beyond the physically obvious.

Don't get me wrong, I understand everyone goes through periods of strength and weakness. That's normal life stuff, and it's very reasonable to need to lean on others when the going gets tough. But if it's always that way, one specific friend constantly leaning on another, it's likely that unhealthy habits such as codependency will develop. And that's helpful or desirable to no one.

Nails are sharp. Just one part, though. I call that the business end. It's that part of the nail that makes them effective. The pointed end of the nail is designed as a wedge to get the rest of the nail into the wood when blunt force is applied to the opposing end. Sometimes friends, in order to help each other out, have to use some force and wedge themselves into our lives. Hopefully, it's done carefully and with love. I've experienced times when it's been necessary for a friend to really hammer a point home, and time wasn't a luxury they were afforded. But this tough love approach is rarely needed. In an ideal world, a friend wouldn't create a lot of resistance to helpful support, allowing loving intervention to slide freely and easily into their lives. That doesn't mean it won't hurt going in. When there is resistance, the helping friend should carefully, systematically work their way into the situation. Otherwise, just like being reckless while using a hammer and nail, something might get smashed, someone will get hurt, and dirty words will fly.

Nails are a very common and useful commodity. But sometimes we run up against problems or situations where a nail just isn't the right solution. Nails are not the answer for everything, right? Sometimes we need a specialty item: screws or glue, for example. I can call a friend when I have leaky pipes or need to change the brake pads on my car. I have friends that know how to do that stuff. But if I have a water-main burst, or my engine dies, I'm going to need to call someone with more experience and expertise. If I'm feeling down, friends are great sources of encouragement, but sometimes my emotions get so complicated that I need a professional to step in. Look … I get it. People like me who struggle with a severe mental illness know the pain a friend may be feeling firsthand. And, because we understand this pain and have developed or learned coping skills, we know what works for us. But we have to realize and admit the limitations we have to offer. We've got to acknowledge what we can and cannot do. This type of gut-level honesty is another of the great characteristics of a quality friend.

Sometimes nails need to be removed. There are a few ways to go about this. We can use the claw of our hammer to pull it out, or we can try to hammer the nail in further to get it out of the way. Another option is to break the nail off at the contact point with the wood. Similarly, sometimes friendships have to end. Quite often, friendships end naturally; people move away, change schools, jobs, or churches. Lots of times a nail will just break on its own. It wears away with time. The loss of a friendship is hard. It can be even more difficult and painful when a friendship needs to be severed intentionally. Later in the book, I will discuss reasons this happens and methods for how to go about doing it. Chances are, this is something we've all experienced. Ending a friendship is tough business.

*You*tilization

For your next exercise, I want you to make a list of all your friends in your journal. These are people that you'd have a game night with or enjoy going to a bar and getting a nice cold chocolate milk with. After you've got your list, go find a nail for each of those people. Twelve friends = twelve nails.

Wanna go even deeper?

Take a second to reflect in your journal about the similarities between a nail and friendship. Ask yourself questions like: What would I use a nail for? If you don't have any nails around the house, ask yourself why not. What would you like to do with your friends? And if you feel like you don't have any friends, why not? Journal your thoughts down.

CYBER-BONDS

Technology has become such an integral part of our daily routine, especially in terms of building and maintaining relationships. That's why I think it's important to address this very unique topic.

Throughout history, friends and family have lived and traveled together in tight-knit communities. I've got this friend, his name is Ruben. We've been friends for about fifteen years. It started when he was dating my wife's friend. After a while, Ruben lost his home and needed a place to crash. I was like, "Dude, my house!" A lot of video games were played when he lived with us. Then he moved out to get married, and now lives in another state. Whether it be snail mail or email, the only way he and I are able to connected is through technology. And that's hard. But why is it hard? Why is the distance such a big deal, especially with all of the communication options we have these days?

When we care about someone, putting distance between us and them, regardless of the available technology, is still really, really difficult. When you care about someone, you want to know what they're up to. You want to be involved in their lives.

In the introduction to the third tool, I talked about the nail and how it represented friendship. It's a very basic bond. It requires physical contact. But we are not always able to physically connect with friends for various reasons, including distance, time, money, health, and yes, even a global pandemic. This lack of in person connection creates countless obstacles for our mental health and leads to people relying almost entirely on technology to do friendship. So how do we use technology in a healthy way to maintain and grow deepening relationships, and what areas of caution should we be aware of? I've got a few ideas. Let's start with a general understanding that **we can do this** despite the challenges.

There is a force that creates bonds and requires no physical contact. It is a technological alternative to traditional ways of bringing two things together, and it gives us a lot more flexibility in how we do it. It allows us to create a very secure bond and disengage the bond quickly. The technology I am referring to is magnetism.

There are lots of things we can do with magnets. They're used to secure doors, lift cars, and even aid in seeing inside the human body as is the case with MRI scanning machines. Magnets are a remarkable form of technology that often get overlooked. Consider the magnets on your fridge. I've got about ten of them holding up Christmas cards and expired coupons. They bond those important (or not so important) reminders to our refrigerator because there is something we want to remember. That is one of the *huge* advantages of technology and friendship. Technology helps us remember! I get reminders on my phone about friend's birthdays, parties, events, etc. I'm able to create reminders on my phone so that I can ask my friends questions or check in on them if I know they've had something happen, good or bad, that would necessitate a little bit more attention.

For hundreds of years, people were limited to using hand-written correspondence to keep in touch with loved ones. This was, and still is, a very meaningful form of technology that combines our intellectual and artistic talents as we write sentences, draw letters with ink, and draw pictures both figuratively and literally. When the telephone became commonplace in the home, friends were able to connect instantaneously, allowing us to lounge around the house, although connected by a cord to the wall, while having conversations. Inflections in voices could be heard, and so a lot of communication depended not only on the words someone said—as was the case with letters, but also on the tone of voice.

Now, with the advent of the internet, communication has become something way more interesting. And by interesting, I mean both really great and utterly disastrous. The internet has become the dominating force in how we interact with our friends. That interaction—and what I want us to focus on here—is called cyber-friendship: relationships made and kept online. I've got serious questions and concerns about this whole idea of cyber-friends. Is it good or bad? Let's explore the concept.

There are three main terms I will be using in this section that you may be unfamiliar with: cyber-bonds, cyber-friends, and hardstuffification. A cyber-bond is the invisible force that holds friendships together using technology. There are two types of cyber-bonds: absolute and partial. Absolute cyber-bonds are those bonds between friends that exist only online. Partial cyber-bonds are those bonds between friends that rely significantly on online interaction but also have an element of in person aspect to them. Cyber-bonds are not static though. People are constantly in transition. Let's say you had a friend growing up that lived next door. Maybe the two of you met at a nearby park and loved to sit on the swing set. Chances are, this childhood friend is no longer a neighbor. Maybe you stay in touch via Facebook Messenger. This relationship has transitioned from non-cyber-bond to absolute cyber-bond. If, in time, you both start hanging out together while maintaining the online connection, then it becomes a partial-cyber-bond relationship. Most of us today are in partial-cyber-bond relationships.

Cyber-friends are the result of cyber-bonds. These are the people being brought together through the internet.

What in the world is hardstuffification? This is a highly technical term (I just made up) used to describe things that make our lives easier, and at the same time, well, harder. Friendship is such a hardstuffificated subject, and nothing hardstuffificates it more than computers and everything we can do with them.

Cyber-friends are a new beast ... or are they? What makes a cyber-friend any different from a pen pal? You remember pen pals, don't you? This was a person you typically never met, or maybe met only once, but communicated with almost entirely through the mail. Are cyber-friendships and pen pals basically the same thing? In some sense I guess they are, but there are significant differences at play here: speed, accessibility, and content. Conversations between cyber-friends happen a million times faster than those with pen pals. Sharing information, asking questions, making requests, providing answers or links to answers, and the ability to share multimedia are all happening at the unique speed of your internet router.

It's one thing for a kid to go off and mail a letter to someone, or to sneak down to the kitchen and call a friend in the middle of the night. But now we have the ability to communicate with anyone in the world virtually at the speed of light, anywhere from the living room to the toilet. From desktops, tablets, phones and watches, to the vehicles we drive, and even our refrigerators, we are being connected to the greater world in a way that is unprecedented. It's important, because of this ease of accessibility, that people with cyber-friends maintain balance. If all you have are cyber-friends but you are perfectly capable of getting out into the natural world and having in person relationships, then I propose you are not living a balanced lifestyle and need to make some changes.

Cyber-dating should also proceed with a huge amount of caution. It's becoming quite common to meet someone online and use that as a way to connect with another person romantically. I've seen these go well, and I've seen them go VERY badly. I can't stress the need for caution loudly enough in these pages, so please just picture me on my knees begging you to be very careful when beginning romantic relationships online. One really good thing about cyber-dating is that it will usually make its way into real life. Once you've connected with them in person, make sure you take a decent amount of time to get to know this new side of them before you make any lifelong commitments. The person you see on the screen is not the whole person you will see when you finally meet them. They may be completely open and honest with you about who they are while chatting online, but there is still a barrier to getting to know them that cannot be breached without some form of in person connection. Wait to make any long-term commitments to anyone until you've had the opportunity to meet in person and get to know each other face to face.

Cyber-bonds can actually give us some idea of how a person is doing socially and emotionally. A study done in 2008, found that people with low self-esteem revealed that online communication actually improved their confidence levels because they didn't have to deal with the awkward nuances of non-verbal communication

(Ando & Sakamoto, 2008). This confidence goes a long way in helping them build face to face relationships. On the other hand, someone with high self-esteem had increased social anxiety when the number of cyber-friends increased. Not surprisingly, the lonelier a person feels in their family relationships, the more likely they are to have more cyber-friends and vice versa. The more cyber-friends a person has, the more likely a person is to be lonely in their family.

It is important to always be somewhat guarded when making friends anywhere you go, but especially online. One of the key things to do is set boundaries for yourself. I call them my rules. Actually take the time to write them out! I'm not telling you what rules to make; figure that out for yourself, but then stick with them. Please be sure to limit your interaction online and don't, for heaven's sake, believe everything you see or read. This technological platform makes putting our best foot forward and holding back any of our flaws super-easy. These flaws may be as innocent as a mole under the right ear, or as problematic as predatory tendencies.

Here is a list of Joe-suggested online boundaries:

1. Nothing good happens after midnight.

2. Create limits to conversations with the sex to which you are attracted.

3. Don't give out personal information.

4. If something feels off or wrong, it probably is.

I think a lot of good can come from online friendships but try to remember to take everything in moderation.

*You*tilization

Grab your journal and write about how technology has changed throughout your lifetime. What are some of the benefits and drawbacks to this new way of living?

Wanna go even deeper?

Contact an older relative and ask them the same question: How has technology affected your friendships throughout your life? Record the conversation if possible. Having these types of meaningful interactions are precious. I did a report on my grandparents and still have the recorded conversation some ten years later. They are both gone now, and so I cherish the recording.

THE LONELINESS CRISIS

When do you feel loneliest? For me, there is one common event that makes me feel lonely even thinking about it. Wedding receptions. I love going to weddings. I'm the sort of guy who gets all mushy and emotional during the vows. But after the wedding, when the party starts, I'm a fish out of water. And would you like to know what makes it even worse? I feel so lonely surrounded by a ton of happy people. Argh! My wife and I have devised a strategy for dealing with this that we've found to be fairly successful. But before I share our little secret with you, I'd like you to know a little bit more about this very serious crisis happening all around the world.

One of the most troubling mental health issues facing people today is loneliness. It seems like such a personal problem, doesn't it? It's a *me* issue. I cause it. I have to fix it. But it's more than just an individual's problem. Leaders in corporations and even national governments are taking notice. It's gotten serious enough for the U.K. to create a Minister for Loneliness (MOL) position in 2018. Tracey Crouch, MOL, says, "Nobody should feel alone or be left with no one to turn to. Loneliness is a serious issue that affects people of all ages and backgrounds and it is right that we tackle it head on (Prime Minister's Office, 2018)."

Is it possible to feel lonely when you have friends? Of course. As I mentioned earlier, I often feel lonely when I am in a packed room. Let me ask you this: Which scenario would you feel lonelier in—being in a packed room full of strangers or friends? It depends, right? If I am in a room full of strangers, it may not really bother me. These are people I don't know or have little, if any, emotional connection with. If I am in a packed room with friends, with people I am deeply, emotionally invested in, the scenario changes drastically. Let's go back to the Mental Health Scale to evaluate this a little more.

If I am at a zero or below on the MHS and am in a room full of friends, more than likely I'm probably feeling lonely. Why? Because there are people all around me that I care about, and I can't possibly connect with every one of them. If I don't connect with everybody, that means someone gets left out. My M.O. is to find a corner to hide in and cover my eyes with a book or behind my phone. The last thing I want to see are people pitying me for the struggle *I think* they think I'm having. Isolating myself keeps me from getting caught up in how I see really complicated social interactions happening all around me. If I am above a zero on the MHS, the scenario changes and loneliness becomes less of an issue. In that situation I'm good, unless something triggers me to drop to a zero or below. And then loneliness and I get to spend some more quality time together.

Friendship, this nurturing of our souls, this connecting of ourselves to someone else, is vitally important. When someone talks about not being lonely for the rest of their lives, they are usually talking about marriage. Marriage is a big commitment. We all need someone to trust, to make us laugh, to cry with us, to bear each other's burdens. And yet, the first year of marriage is usually one of the loneliest times in our lives. Oftentimes people turn to marriage to solve their loneliness issues, only to find out that it complicates them even more. Intimate relationships such as marriage are not a solution to loneliness. Deep, loving relationships work better when expectations are low and commitment and determination is high.

What is a good way to deal with loneliness? One strategy is to identify self-pity as soon as possible. When I feel lonely, many times it's because I've felt rejected. I think, "What's wrong with me?" or "Why don't people want to spend time with me?" And then I start to dwell on those thoughts, especially when I feel like I've been forgotten. "I guess I am just easy to forget," is a common thought I have. Pay careful attention to your thoughts and personal narrative when you feel lonely so that you don't become bitter. It's helpful to recognize and tell ourselves that our friends are doing their best. Trying to get attention or to convince people to focus on us through self-pity is a nasty, addictive drug and is hazardous to your emotional health. Nine times out of ten, people will get what they want through complaining and whining. That's why self-pity is such an issue. It is the root of a much larger sickness: external validation achieved through manipulation and guilt. Instead of self-pity, talk to the person you felt left out by. Be understanding. Be forgiving. If your friend forgot about you, they'll be thankful you talked to them. If they've been intentionally ignoring you, then you'll be thankful, in time, that you figured this out and can decide on some healthy next steps sooner rather than later. True friends really value up-fronted-ness. It's not always easy to give or receive at first. It's that way for everyone. But it's something I've found to be a really healthy component to good friendships.

If you're feeling lonely, it really is up to you to take action. You're the only person who can do anything about it. Talk to your therapist, doctor, and friends, and let them know this is something you're struggling with. Addressing the problem head on is the best way to get on a path toward healthy emotional independence. Oh, and the way I deal with loneliness at wedding receptions? I have begun to bring things to do. My wife and I have noticed that the loneliness sets in when the eating is over, right when the dancing starts. That's when I kiss my wife goodbye and head to the car for a little *me* time until she's ready to go or the reception is over. I can't stress enough how great this plan has worked for us!

I can't wait for you to get to the next three exciting topics: starting friendships, keeping friends, and should a friendship end. Each one of these subjects needs to be considered very carefully and can do one of two things: create tremendous roadblocks toward mental wellness or promote mental well-being. But first, let's *You*tilize what we have discussed in this chapter.

*You*tilization

Think about times in the past when you've felt lonely. Are there any similarities? It wasn't hard to figure out that loneliness was an issue for me at wedding receptions. How about you? And what strategy can you put into action when loneliness creeps in? Yes, I'd like you to either write about it in your journal or talk about it with a loved one.

Wanna go even deeper?

One of the easiest things to forget when you feel lonely is that there are other people in your world who feel lonely too. It's easy to forget because loneliness is not a very popular topic of conversation. I often tell people who feel lonely to reach out to people who may also be feeling lonely. Search out these people. Write them a letter (yes, a physical letter), and mail it. One of the best ways I've dealt with loneliness is to find other lonely people to be vulnerable with. And what happens when you get a bunch of lonely people together who are battling loneliness? They become less lonely.

STARTING FRIENDSHIPS

The Best Friend You Didn't Know You Had

You are the best friend you didn't know you had; and if you're not, you should be. If you want to be a good friend, if you want to start and maintain healthy, nurturing friendships, then you need to start with being your own best friend. There are a few really great tips I want to share with you to help you be your own best friend, but first let me start by telling you why it's so important.

Want to be a better friend to your friends? Start by being your own best friend. Maybe you feel worn out and overwhelmed trying to maintain the friends you already have. One of the really cool things about being your own best friend is that you never have to get dressed up or even leave your house to spend time with yourself. You have the luxury of friend time 24/7 with that gorgeous person you see in the mirror! But for some of us, that might be the problem. We look in the mirror—either literally or figuratively—and don't like what we see. In fact, we can't even look at ourselves because we are so overwhelmed with the flaws and unmet personal expectations that we see every time we do. I get it. If you're anything like me, you are viciously critical of that person who is constantly looking back at you. You're not alone. I am absolutely convinced that the more you get to know yourself and the more you allow yourself to be you, the more you will like who you are.

Wouldn't it be great if the people and things we are constantly surrounded with were the people and things that we felt the most connected to? But proximity doesn't breed intimacy. In fact, it can repel it. You can go through life being happily miserable with yourself and live a very long life. You wouldn't be the first, and you certainly won't be the last. BUT, wouldn't it be nice if that guy or gal you look at in the mirror every day was someone you cared very deeply for? I'm not just talking about "care" as a decision. I'm talking about a genuine feeling of deep love and concern for yourself. It's so possible and so very important. It's what I desperately want for you and me! Take a look at these really great ideas to help us get there.

Listen to Yourself

A great place to start being your own best friend is to listen to yourself. There is an inner part of you that is constantly trying to help. But this can be hard and even confusing because which "inner-you" do you listen to? Maybe you've got a part of you that says," Don't take chances ... you'll get hurt." Or the opposite," Take all the chances or you'll regret it if you don't." That's what it's like for me at least. I can't seem to find a consensus in my own brain. This disagreement isn't necessarily a bad thing, although it can feel frustrating. This is the inner-you that's trying to help you survive and be all that you can be. This inner-you has been developing your whole life, slowly gaining influence and volume with each decision you make. It's the inner-you that has taught you how to deal with and understand how the world works and what you need to do about it. I want you to develop a routine to really listen to that inner-you. Find a comfortable and quiet spot to sit. The places that work best for me are a cemetery, the secluded shoreline of a river or lake when weather permits, or curled up with my journal and a favorite beverage on my living room recliner. Listen to what is going on inside of you. Record your thoughts in your journal. While you're listening, I want you to also think about what you're feeling. Think about your emotions (an example of mindfulness for all you CBT/DBT geeks out there). The more you listen to yourself, the more you'll trust this inner-you. And, with time, the more you listen and trust yourself, the more comfortable you will be in your own skin, and I'm confident that you will grow to really like who you are.

Take Care of Yourself

I want you to change the way you think about yourself. I want you to consider yourself on a hierarchal list of friends as friend numero uno. There is a good reason for this, but you've got to give me a minute. First things first. Before I get into what taking care of yourself is, or better explain what taking care of yourself can look like, let's first consider what NOT taking care of yourself looks like. One of the first things that happens when you stop taking care of yourself is you start to let yourself go. Wait. Doesn't that sound a little redundant? But let me explain what I mean.

Have you ever seen one of those end-of-the-world type movies where a plague or aliens have destroyed all but a few human beings on the planet? The survivors wander around major cities that have been overrun by wildlife and vegetation. It's weird to see big cities like New York or Los Angeles completely abandoned and taken over by Mother Nature. That is what I mean by letting go. It means not regularly caring for yourself. You pay less attention to your health. You don't watch what you eat. You splurge more, spending time and money on things that are harmful to your mind or body. I tend to stop showering and brushing my teeth. When you don't care about you, putting others before yourself sounds nice. Who doesn't want to give their friends the best they have. In reality though, that "best" you're giving them isn't really that great because all that's left, all they're getting, is barely enough to coat the bottom of your emotional barrel.

I've been there before. Feeling emotionally drained, like my soul is all dried out. It's left me spending a good chunk of my time playing emotional catch-up and, just like with credit card debt, always paying for my past pains with my present strength. It's an unhealthy way to live. When does it stop? How does it stop? It stops when I decide enough is enough and actually *choose* to stop. But choosing is easier said than done. That's why we need connections. That's why we need friends.

Caring for yourself is even a foundational teaching found in the Bible. Jesus taught people to love others the way you love yourself. He didn't mean that we should love others and not take care of ourselves. He was telling us to evaluate how well we take care of ourselves and use that as the foundation or starting point for taking care of others. God wants you to think about how incredibly fantastic you are, and then treat others the same way. So, that *choosing thing* I just mentioned can start with choosing to consider how you want to treat the people you love, and then start treating yourself the same way. Loving yourself is good practice for being the loving friend you want to be.

The problem I have, and maybe you do too, is that Jesus' words, "Love your neighbor as yourself," get all messed up in my head. When I'm not properly taking care of myself, his words become "Love your neighbor as much as you think you should, which is definitely a lot more than you currently are, and most certainly more than you could ever love yourself."

How have I taken such a straightforward teaching from Jesus and jumbled it all up? Well, to be honest, it's not something I've done alone. I grew up in a church-culture that taught service and sacrifice with absolutely no mention of personal boundaries and self-care/awareness. Many churches are starting to do an about-face to this type of leadership style. My church in particular takes very good care of volunteers and deeply values their emotional wellbeing. But back in the day, people were expected to lay down their lives for the cause of Christ because God promises not to give us more than we can bear (feel free to read more about this "promise" in 1 Corinthians 10, verse 13). Can you see the dangerous inference there? If a person overdoes it and gets burned out or has some moral failure as a result of doing too much, who's to blame? Certainly not God. And definitely not the church. The *obvious* assumption is that they were acting outside of God's will and trying to do too much, probably out of pride. "They did this to themselves."

A major problem is that there is a lot of truth in what they are saying. Just enough truth to raise doubt in the burnt-out individual. What often gets ignored is that the organizational church pressures people into doing things in the name of God while taxing people to their emotional and physical limits without providing guidance to help people determine what appropriate limits are. The more people ignore their own needs (i.e. denying themselves), the more they give the power and authority not over to Jesus, but to the institution of organized religion. How often do you hear leadership telling you to rest more? Jesus certainly rested a lot! One of his most vulnerable times, when he was fasting for forty days, he was alone in the wilderness. He separated himself from everyone else knowing how important, and probably, how difficult this period would be for his mind and body. When I take care of myself by showering regularly, taking my meds, exercising, and getting the appropriate amount of rest, I often feel guilty for not doing enough for others. I've come to realize that I will never do enough to satisfy that echoing, nagging voice in the back of my head telling me to do more for others.

So ... what can we do? A good start is to acknowledge our feelings. Put a label on them. This will help us do what needs to be done next ... which is to ask for help. And keep asking for help until we actually *feel* helped. Don't settle for anything else. Don't judge yourself for getting help when others say you've gotten enough. We are all just trying to muddle through life, and no one else will ever walk in our shoes.

If you've ever been on an airplane, then you've heard the flight attendant's speech about fastening your seatbelts when the light is on, identifying where the emergency exits are, and the part when they tell you your seat is a floatation device?! Am I the only one that's ever been tempted to take the seat apart and look at it? And then they show you how to use the oxygen mask. If the cabin loses pressure, it falls like a venomous snake in a bad horror film, but you are supposed to put it on and breathe normally?! Only after you have yours on are you supposed to help the person next to you. Airlines know the benefit of taking care of yourself first. Take one from their playbook, get yourself to a safe emotional place, then you can think clearly enough to help someone else. It's really hard to take your friends to a place of emotional safety without knowing the way or having been their yourself. So find your way, and then take others with you.

If you're worried that you're being selfish when you don't help someone else first, ask your spouse or ask a friend. Sit them down and talk to them about your concerns, and then ask them for their honest, un-watered-down opinion. If they say, "Yeah, you're being pretty selfish," then listen to that, but don't own it … yet. Talk to more than one person to find a consensus. My suggestion is a minimum of three people. If three people out of five are telling you you're selfish then, well, let me put it this way: If a person calls you a horse, you can laugh it off and walk away. If two people say you're a horse, just shrug and walk it off. But if three people call you a horse, then it may be time to go buy a saddle. More likely than not, you're just stuck in your head, living in fear of something that needs to be worked out in therapy. So a good third choice is to rescue yourself before you try rescue anyone else.

*You*tilization

Take yourself out on a date. That's right. Get dressed up. Maybe buy yourself some flowers. Get that favorite dessert you love. Don't forget the smell-well (my kids word for cologne or perfume). Just go. Enjoy you!

Wanna go even deeper?

While you are out enjoying yourself, take your journal along. While you're at dinner or sitting at the movie theatre, make some notes about the things you like. What things stick out to you? What things don't appeal to you? This is all part of getting to know yourself. And after the day is done, reflect on it. What was easy? What was awkward or difficult? What would you do differently next time? And then, schedule the next date and make any changes you thought of.

Like Yourself

When I'm having a bad day and tell someone I don't like myself, it usually means two things: First, as confusing as it may sound, I don't mean I don't like myself. Instead, it's just really hard to care, and I wish I didn't have to, so I pretend like I don't matter because I don't know what else to do. Secondly, it means that I want that person I am talking to to tell me something specific they like about me. That's why I'm telling them. Do you like yourself? This is a legit question that I ask myself quite often. Here's the deal ... I find myself liking the person I want to be. But unfortunately, I rarely like myself where I am. Why am I so unlikeable to myself? I was listening to a podcast that shared this quote from Chuck Palahniuck's book *Invisible Monster*, "When we don't know who to hate, we hate ourselves." Maybe you can relate, maybe not, but this seems to be one of the biggest battles I face that is directly linked to my mental illness: I don't like myself.

Let's look at the connection between liking yourself and self-friendship; the two are closely linked. How can I go from how I currently feel about myself to actually liking or loving myself? Here's the thing: when I like myself, which does happen from time to time, it's hard for me to imagine *not* liking myself. I've tried. I just can't get myself to understand why I'm so hard on myself. But when I don't like who I am, it's really hard to admit that I have ever liked me. It's like someone turned off the emotional lights in my head. To be honest, this idea of liking myself seems completely foreign and a little bit silly to me, but at that the same time, absolutely imperative. We need to retrain our brains and learn to like ourselves.

Here are a few practical ideas to move you in the right direction:

- <u>Spend more time with yourself.</u> Notice I said *with* yourself not *by* yourself. For me there is a distinction. When I'm by myself, I tend to think of isolation and boredom. When you say you are "with someone," it sounds intimate; that you are in a position to get to know or are getting to know someone. If I said I was standing by someone famous, you would never assume that person and I were close friends or even acquainted. Being *by* someone is a physical proximity. But if I said I was *with* a famous person, then you may see the deeper connection. I want you to make that deeper connection with yourself!

- <u>Date yourself.</u> Take yourself out to dinner and a movie. Experiment with restaurants and foods as well as different genres of movies. Expose yourself to new surroundings- in legally acceptable ways please—to see if there is something you'd like that you've never tried before. Did you dress up? You should! Check yourself out in the mirror. Maybe even let someone else know how good you look.

- <u>Whisper sweet nothings to yourself.</u> I already know you talk to yourself, so why not encourage yourself when you do something right. Send yourself "You're awesome" texts or voicemails.

- <u>Have some fun.</u> One of the best things you can do to be a friend is to go have some fun. This may be hard to do when you go out alone, but who says you have to take yourself out all by yourself. Maybe you could get a bunch of people together who are taking themselves out and do a double or triple date. Let loose. Footloose. Drink an extra pint or two of chocolate milk. Enjoy yourself!

- <u>Hold yourself.</u> Just wrap your sweet arms around yourself and give yourself some lovin'.

- <u>Give yourself a gift.</u> Seriously, when have you ever wrapped a present for yourself? Don't open it right away. Set a specific date and time for you to receive it. There's a good chance you'll forget about it and be surprised one day.

- <u>Acknowledge where you are in life</u>. Have you ever had a moment when it just clicked: "I'm an adult?" Frightening, right? This happened to me a few years back. One day I was hit with the realization that I could go out and buy a box of Lucky Charms anytime I wanted to. I'm free to want what I want! What a novel idea. So, give yourself some quality time. My wife does this really well. She loves to get her nails done, go to the movies by herself, get her hair cut, or sit in the tub with bath salts, a glass of wine, and Netflix. Enjoy where you're at and who you are!

How do we begin to make ourselves a priority? If you remember back in the sections about journaling, I mentioned my four major life priorities: God, Health, Family, and Me. Being kind and generous to yourself every day is a big part of being your own friend. Through therapy, I've learned to balance my wants and needs. The key word there is balance!

The main idea here, and the whole purpose of Broken People, is to remind you that you are not alone and to take care of yourself. When you take really good care of yourself, not only will you be in a better position to care for other people, but you'll want to care for other people because you just feel so awesome! Take one or two of the things I've mentioned above and start doing them today. It won't be easy. The best changes usually happen gradually, but they are really awesome when they do. And for goodness sake, please enjoy yourself.

*You*tilization

Your next task is to take some of the ideas I mentioned today, or create some of your own and schedule them on your phone or in your calendar. If there is anything I learned while publishing this book, it's that if I don't write something down, it probably won't happen.

Wanna go even deeper?

It's really hard to change how we think until we change what we do. Make a list of all of your best qualities. If you can't think of any, ask a friend or family member. Once you have those *written down*, set an alarm for three times in the next twenty-four hours to go stand in front of a mirror, look yourself in the eye, and say those things to yourself with as much passion and self-love as possible. Seriously though, be a little creepy about it.

The Ingredients of a Good Friend

School had already been underway for a couple of weeks. It was my senior year at a small, private high school in Dearborn Heights, Michigan. A friend stopped me in the doorway to our homeroom at the beginning of the day to make a serious request. She wanted me to know that there was a new guy in our class, that a few girls were already saying he was good looking, and that she thought I would be a good person to befriend him. She was concerned that this guy would be drawn into the "cool-kid" group and be tainted. I was flattered to be considered for such an important mission: deterring this guy from the reprehensible in-crowd. But I also felt a little worried that I wouldn't be effective in my efforts. When I went into the classroom, I sought out this debonair fellow and found him sitting in the middle seat of the middle row. "This guy? This is going to be easier than I thought." I sat next to him, struck up a conversation, and thus began a friendship that continues today, some twenty-seven years later.

This guy I met that day in school, Adam, has been instrumental in forming the person I am today. I think and hope he would say the same about me. Friends do that, don't they?

Unfortunately, there aren't many resources that give us insight on how to find, choose, and be friends. There are, however, good examples of friendship in many fiction stories. In *Of Mice and Men*, the odd friendship of

George and Lennie grew out of a sense of responsibility to Lennie's aunt. In *The Lord of the Rings*, a friendship developed between Frodo and Sam because of a greater good that needed to be accomplished.

Because people have different wants and needs, there is no perfect recipe for making friends. Friendships are as unique as a fingerprint: no two are the same.

In this chapter, I'll use this recipe analogy to try to draw out some of the key ingredients of a quality friend. One of the unique aspects of me talking about cooking is that I am not the cook in our household. Melissa, my wife, fills that role. So this should be interesting, and quite possibly fraught with errors, much as my baking typically is (just ask my kids about my infamous spaghetti burgers). But let's find those errors together.

I generally see recipes (and this may cause some of you professionals out there to cringe) as a list of suggestions. Options really, to be taken or left out at the cook's discretion. Of course, this will change the overall outcome, but that's where *you* uniqueness and style really shine. So I challenge you do to the same with the list I'm about to present to you. Take it as a skeleton of sorts, for you to add to or subtract from based upon your personal preferences.

Many times, friendships are made by accident. People gather together in a place, strike up a conversation, and hit it off. Have you ever wondered what caused a person to experiment with something, eat it, and then decide to introduce it to others as a food source? Take milk for example. Who decided to try the creamy excretions from one of a cow's multiple … nipples? How did it ever cross someone's mind to consider putting these things in their mouth? My guess? Necessity. People were hungry, and they did what they had to to find food wherever it could be found. Personally, I believe this is why my kids enjoy Taco Bell. I think friendships are often born from necessity as well. You work with what you've got. What's immediately around you.

If you haven't already noticed, I do things a bit differently. I typically seek out people like a bug seeks out a windshield, except hopefully without the disastrous outcome. I started doing this a while ago, because I heard somewhere that you are the average of your ten closest friends. This is not something I want left to chance. So ask yourself, "Self, who do you want to be five or ten years from now?" Then seek out people who fit the bill. People who are like the person you want to be.

There are a lot of buzzwords out there that are commonly associated with the makings of a good friend. In recipes you may have flour, sugar, vanilla extract, and oil; in friendships you commonly hear love, respect, trust, and selflessness. These are not things you want to ignore, no matter how boring or often you hear them. Removing just one of these key ingredients will lead you to a bitter experience. My daughter made a couple pumpkin pies for Thanksgiving in 2018. This is my favorite pie and one of my favorite foods in the world. I was getting out of the shower at the time everyone started eating it and heard their gasps. I could just barely make out that she'd forgotten the sugar. I decided to come out of the shower and play dumb (which is something I do a lot), request a piece of pumpkin pie, and pretend to eat it as if nothing was wrong. I knew I would be closely watched when that first bite entered my mouth, and I did everything within my power to keep a straight face. Success. I made it until about the third bite, refusing eye contact with anyone else in the room, eyes watering, until I had to give up and run for the waste bin. Those traits above … love, respect, trust, and selflessness … you really can't go without them. You can try to fake a friendship for a time, but it will leave your eyes watering and a nasty taste in your mouth.

On to a more interesting friendship characteristic: imperfection. This is one of the most important things I look for in a friendship. Let's face it: no one is perfect. And if I have to look super hard to find your imperfections, something is terribly wrong. Why is imperfection such an important trait to me? It gives me something to relate to. If I have a friend that doesn't understand defeat and struggle, how will they ever understand me? I've had several friendships where they were not willing to share their pains and problems with me. When this happens, it doesn't necessarily mean we can't be friends, but it does limit the depth of it. And the depth of friendship is ultimately a two-person decision. It takes two to tango.

Another note about perfection: it is typically a relative term, especially in the culinary world. I may not make the recipe exactly the way it's written down, but only I know my likes and dislikes. I'm not going to put certain things in foods if I don't like them. For example, the Whopper comes with mayo, but I can't describe to you the utter devastation I feel when I order my burger with lettuce, cheese, and tomatoes through the drive-thru, only to find out that it has mayonnaise contaminating it. It literally ruins the whole experience for me.

I skip a lot of ingredients in recipes that are not to my taste. I also skip over a lot of really great people as friends. And that's ok. Follow your heart. I'm not drawn to loud, overly confident people. I don't enjoy grabbing a few beers at the local watering hole. I love connecting with friends on a deeper level while helping them complete a project around their house or on a leisurely stroll along a river walk or through a cemetery. It's just how I roll. Once I was able to come to grips with that, being a good friend and finding good friends has been a heck of a lot easier.

Here's another ingredient I have found to be important as I pursue friends: acceptance. I'm just as guilty as the next person, changing who I am to get people to like me. It's extremely frustrating because it's really hard to figure out what the other person's tastes are and then to try to adapt yourself to fit their expectations. When you have to change who you are to be with someone else, the relationship is destined for failure unless you change back to who you really are ... which is complicated, right? Instead of disguising who I am under the cloak of who I think I should be, I've learned that I am a pretty great guy and worth having people in my life who like me for me. And so are you! But this leads to a more frustrating problem. I've had a heck of a time trying to figure out who I am so that I could be that person. And here is what I found: you cannot find yourself by looking. I know, I've tried. You can only find yourself by living. I do what I do, live in line with my passions and the opportunities that are before me, and then, through those events, I learn who I am. I'm learning to be patient and to let who I am develop over time. Then I am able to reflect on who that is. This one change has blown the door open for deeper, more meaningful friendships!

One Saturday, I volunteered to make food for an event at my church. They asked for soups, and so I decided to make my favorite: chicken noodle. I followed the directions in the recipe as closely as I was comfortable but left out things that I didn't particularly care for. Long story short, it looked like mush by the time the event rolled around. But people tried it and most seemed to like it! One of my pastors even came up to tell me that it was her favorite dish. Acceptance doesn't always mean that you like everything about another person, it just means that you acknowledge the differences and maybe find a way to appreciate them. Anyway, it's those differences that make us unique and add a pinch of spice into our lives, don't you think?

There's not a ton of stuff you can read about defining friendships, but I'd highly suggest you check out Dale Carnegie's *How to Win Friends and Influence People* and Aristotle's description of the three types of friendships in his Nichomachean Ethics work. The important thing is to keep experimenting with the recipes. Find what you like, identify what you don't. Find those people you like, limit your exposure to those you don't. Go on. It's ok to be picky.

*You*tilization

For your next adventure, I'd like you to make a cake (sure, brownies or cupcakes are fine) and take it to a friend. If the thought of making a cake gives you hives... go buy one. But seriously, try to make it! Get the cake mix, the eggs, and make it happen. And as you work, think about the ingredients that I mentioned in this chapter that go into making a good friendship. Are there a couple I missed? After you've delivered the cake, email me. I'd love to hear about your experience. Joe@broken-people.org

Wanna go even deeper?

Think about the ingredients and actions that went into making the cake. Do these remind you of certain aspects of friendship? For example, cracking an egg might remind you that some friends have a hard, outer shell that you have to get through to find the gooey goodness inside. What other things about the baking process remind you of friendship. Write these down in your journal.

Making Friends as Adults

Am I the only person who finds that it's a uniquely different experience making friends as adults versus being kids? It seems a lot harder to me. Why do you think that is? Consider the words that may come to mind when you think of children and friendship: imagination, creativity, play, sleepovers. Now consider the words that come to mind when you think about adults and friends: um ... beer? What happens when we become adults that seems to make friendship so complicated? Whatever the complexity, I think it's important that we acknowledge it exists, and then figure out what in the world to do about it.

One of the things that changed when I became an adult was that I had fewer people telling me what to do. You may think I'm joking with all the laws and bosses and COVID 19 restrictions we've been dealing with as I'm writing this, but when we were kids, we still had all of those things (except the awesome face mask regulations) AND our parents or guardians deciding what we ate, where we slept, what school we went to, and who we hung out with. As adults, we no longer have someone making most of those decisions for us. I think this leads to decision overload, and our brains get clogged with those decisions, and all the responsibilities, information, and options that come along with them (kind of like mental constipation). And between the stress of working a job, paying bills, putting food on the table, and family time, friendship seems to be something that often easily gets sidelined.

Then there are our rule-fences. These are the invisible boundaries that we put up to keep us from making fools of ourselves. They're there so that we look and sound like adults should look and sound. But as kids, isn't that one of the things we avoided? We never called it being foolish, at least I didn't. I called it being silly. When we fall in love, oftentimes people will make a fool of themselves to win the heart of the one they love. A lot of rules exist for rules 'sake alone. I think we should let these go. Here are a few unwritten rules I've found in my life and some ideas about how to break them:

Rule #1. It's childish and weird to ask someone to be your friend.

Whenever I tell myself to not do something because it's weird, it's like an alarm goes off in my head screeching, *"You need to do this! You need to do this!"* I'm learning to run toward weird. This idea is so simple. Why don't we ask people to be friends more often? Here's what I think: It's a fear of perception and rejection. As adults we want to be perceived as having it together, knowing the answers, being winners and independent. Asking for something makes us look needy and weak. Guess what? I'm needy and weak. How about you? And rejection? When you ask for something, in your mind there is at least a fifty-fifty chance that you're going to be rejected.

And when I became an adult, rejection was one of those things that I wanted to be done with. Rejection is a normal part of our childhood; we get cut from the basketball team, friends pick us last to play tag, and parents tell us," No, you may not repel out of your second story window." And so we run from rejection when we become adults. We want to be so close to certainty before we decide to do something that we find ourselves doing very little. Do you see someone you like or you think is cool and want to hang out with them? Go up to them and ask them. And, as you get to know them, and enjoy their company more, ask the question, "You know what, would you like to be my friend?" More than likely they will say something along the lines of, "I already thought we were friends?" But why mince words and leave commitments undone or unsaid. Seal the deal. Take the risk. You'll feel better for it.

Rule #2: Friends shouldn't ask other friends to help with projects.

I didn't think I'd be able to do it, but there it lay. A fifty-foot tree safely brought down by yours truly in my friend's backyard. My friend was concerned that a storm would knock the tree over on the house or the neighbor's fence, so he wanted it gone. I am not an arborist. I'm a FedEx guy. But, one day, my friend Mike called me and asked for help with a dead tree in his backyard. It was a tall tree. And it had a decent width. I was skeptical that we should be doing anything of the sort, so I'm like, "Yeah, let's do it!" So on a Saturday morning, Mike, his dad, and I donned our gloves and prepared for Operation Cut The Tree Down. But things didn't go quite according to plan.

The most fun I have with my friends is when we're doing a project together. If you know someone you think would make a good friend, invite them over to help with something or ask them if they need help doing anything. You'll learn a lot about a person when you work with them toward a common goal. I have a counter-rule to rule #2 that helps me know when it's okay to ask someone for help, whether it's with a project or anything else. I always ask myself, "Self," (because I always start off that way) "would you think it was weird, rude, or odd if they asked you to come over and help with a project?" Obviously if I think it's weird or odd, I'm going to invite them over anyway because that's just what I do. But in regard to being rude, if my answer to myself is no, I don't feel like it'd be rude if they asked for my help, then I give myself the green light to ask them. Projects give you something to keep you busy when awkward silences threaten to rip your soul in two. We've all been there. That quiet moment when no one knows what to say. And then you look into the eyes of your friend and you both know it's really awkward. I hate that! I feel so insecure; like there is something wrong with me. Am I boring this person? These types of things are usually not a one-way street. Embrace the awkward, get rid of rules that limit how you should make and interact with friends, and get out there and make them.

I was very nervous the morning of Operation Cut the Tree Down, but I had a plan. If we got a rope high enough around the tree, I knew we'd be able to guide the fall while it was being cut. I used a string attached to a hammer to get the sturdier rope about sixty percent of the way up. Once I secured a knot at about twenty feet, I waited for the sound of the chainsaw. And waited. And waited. And waited?

Rule #3: Play time is over.

Why have we stopped playing? Maybe you haven't! That's awesome! Here's an idea: Imagine. Create. Play. Have sleepovers. It seems like play was the first thing to go when we became adults. But if anyone needs to play, it's us! We have so many more problems to deal with than kids do which could be solved with a little bit of fun and imagination. We should use our imaginations as we think about our future, to be creative with friends, and to deepen the bond between ourselves and friends and family. Create with your friends. If you have an idea, invite friends along to help out. Let them see who you are through your imagination and ideas. Maybe you'll inspire something in them. Please play with your friends. Grab an old board game and head to the local diner. Shoot hoops, play tennis, or work out together.

Sleepovers: Go camping with friends. Reserve a cabin a couple of hours away and have some friend time.

Friendship hasn't changed. We've changed. Our responsibilities have changed. One of the big responsibilities that affects how we spend our time as adults is having children of our own. As your kids grow, do you play with them? Sure, you're leading them, but you are also becoming friends—a friendship that will reveal itself more solidly when your child has the option to spend time with you or to do something else. I also think it is vitally important for parents to demonstrate healthy friendships to their children. Children, especially at a younger age, idolize their parents. Even as they grow up, the way a parent engages with other people has a huge impact on how they do friendship. Your children watch you intently to learn how to act when they grow up. If you're married, are you treating your spouse like a dear friend? Do you laugh with your friends? Help them out? Allow them to help you out? Talk and debate about larger life issues with care and compassion? As you do friendship, you are also training up a whole other generation of friends to come. How about them apples?

Back to the tree. I was waiting for the buzz of the chainsaw … nada. I went to check out what was going on. No gas. "Where's Mike?" He did the thoughtful thing and went to the neighbors to let them know we were taking down a tree, just in case something happened and it fell on them. When Mike got back, he and his dad were arranging to get the gas. I just wanted to play with the tree. I put on some gloves, went to the rope attached to the tree, and gave it a little tug. *pop!* Tug .... *creeeeeeeek.* Yank!! ......*tiiiiimber!* It fell quickly and safely in the small green knoll known as my friend's backyard. Talk about having fun! I will forever be known as "the guy who pulled down that big tree" to my friend.

*You*tilization

Do you have kids of your own, or maybe a friend that does? Set up a date to take your child or your friend and their kid out for a cola. While you are out, ask the young scholar their opinion about what it takes to find a friend? Ask them how they met their friends, and then to give you some advice how to make your own.

Wanna go even deeper?

Got a project that needs to be done at your house? Does your friend need help with a project they're working on? I always start with the offer. And let them know you are serious, that if they need anything, you're the one they should talk to! If you can't help, you'll let them know. So reach out. Make the ask.

KEEPING FRIENDS

Conflict

"You're a *<insert female reproductive organ here>*." That's the text I got from one of my best friends when I was telling him about an issue I was having at home. He was frustrated with me because I wouldn't handle the problem the way he would handle it … which involved yelling and "manning up," whatever that meant. His comment stung. I've never had a friend insult me like that before. I sank into my bed where I'd been propped up, cradled my phone, and stared dumbly through glassy eyes at the text.

What are you supposed to do when something like this happens with a friend? Before I do anything, I feel. That's pretty much how I do everything. And the feeling I usually have is insecurity. "There must be something wrong with me. I feel so messed up and broken." After the feelings, I usually do one of two things, or both: I apologize for causing the conflict or I somehow find myself agreeing with them. It didn't take much to convince me that I was the person in the wrong. After all, I just knew my existence was a mistake, and so all of my opinions must be mistakes as well.

How about rejection? What do you do when someone rejects your opinions or ideas? For me, I have this twisted belief that when someone rejects my thoughts or ideas, they are rejecting me. I'm not sure where this theory came from, but it's been around my whole life. So, what do we do with all this ... stuff?

Fortunately for me, because of therapy and good-old-fashioned growing up, I've become more honest about my opinions and how I feel. I've learned that relationships go much deeper than the issues we discuss, and to actually value the disagreements, because when we disagree, we are getting to see and know a part of our friends that makes us different. We are all unique people. And when we find ourselves in conflict with someone we care about, it gives us the golden opportunity, despite those differences, to *choose* to love each other. That *choosing* is the essence of a lasting, deep, and loyal friendship.

Conflict will inevitably happen between friends, but how should we deal with it? The biggest key to unlocking conflict is effective communication. This means speaking and listening effectively. Where do we start? Here are a few tips:

Start by speaking:

- Just kidding, don't speak. Zip it! Whenever you're having a conflict with a friend, it's always good to start by listening to their concern. Don't speak. Listen. What if you and your friend are both reading my book? Who listens first? It doesn't matter! Flip a coin. Draw straws. If it gets to this point, though, it sounds like you both are in a really good place to resolve this conflict and you will listen well when the other is speaking. (Oh, and thanks for buying my book.)

Listen

1. One of the best pieces of advice I've received about what to do when someone is talking to me is that I should be doing one thing and one thing only: listening. Focus on their words. Look into their eyes (don't be creepy about it, though). Don't let there be any doubt that the person has your complete attention and that what they are saying matters to you! There will be times when someone will walk up to you while you're in the middle of a conversation with someone else and want to talk. Unless their hair is on fire, don't break eye contact. Hold up a finger (preferably an appropriate one) to let that person know it'll be a moment before they'll get your attention. I feel the same way about call-waiting. Don't put someone on hold just because someone else is trying to get your attention. This is especially true when there is conflict. When you have a conversation about a disagreement, make sure you talk at a time and in a space that will be quiet and free from

distractions. Parents, let the kids know beforehand if you're going to be having a difficult conversation with someone. Give them some idea of how long it will take and do your best to stick to it. If you end up needing to go a bit longer, take a second during the conversation to step away and give the kids a heads up. Oh, and your cell phone? Please don't hold it in your hand when you're having a serious conversation. Put it in your pocket or set it down. I think we listen better when we are not being distracted by technology.

2. **Actively listen.** This is something that took me some time to get used to. One of the best ways to actively listen is by repeating what was said back to the person who said it. This lets them know you're fully engaged in the conversation, that they are being heard, and helps them to know that you understand what's being said. You may be tempted to paraphrase with a little bit of passive aggressiveness if you don't agree or like what you're hearing. But I hope you'd be wise enough to avoid any type of aggressive response because you see the awesomeness of their willingness to share the conflict with you. Not many people like conflict, and it should be considered high praise for your friend to come and speak to you about it directly.

3. **Listen to what the person is saying, but not just the words.** Listen carefully to the inflections in their voice. This may say more about their fears and feelings than their actual words. Did they get quiet during part of the conversation? Did they mumble a specific word or thought? Maybe this is an aspect of conflict that is hardest for them to share and needs a little bit more love and understanding.

4. **Listen to their body language**. Pay close attention to facial expressions. If they're sitting, are they shaking their knees? Are they touching their face a lot? What they are saying, especially during their visibly anxious moments, may reveal a lot about what they think and feel. What does their posture tell you? Listening to someone should engage more senses than just your ears.

5. **Avoid, at all costs, trying to formulate your own response while your friend is talking.** What that person is saying to you is more important than what you want to say in response to them.

After they have said everything they feel they've needed to say, tell them you want to take some time (length will vary depending on the situation) to think about it before responding, and then:

1. Apologize if you think you're in the wrong.

2. Don't apologize if you don't think you're in the wrong. If you disagree with something the person says, don't pander to your own insecurity by saying you agree with them even when you don't. This is disrespectful to them and to yourself. It is entirely possible that you may disagree with that person but they still could be right. If they are right, you need to apologize or acknowledge that you're wrong despite how you feel. It won't be easy at first, but you'll feel better in the long run.

3. If you are the person addressing the conflict, be honest about it. The longer you let it sit and simmer, the more damage it can do in your heart and mind. Just rip that Band-Aid off. Talk to your friend. They will thank you for it in the long run. And if they don't, you may have just dodged a bullet.

4. Affirm your friend. Make sure your friend understands that you are sharing this with them because you value them.

I don't enjoy conflict, and I'm guessing you don't either. I've gone from being the guy with zero confidence and apologizing even when I thought I was right, to being more honest with my friends about my insecurities while standing up for what I believe to be true. Be honest. Be open. Your friendships will be better, more fulfilling, more fun, and healthier when you are honest with them and yourself.

One last note about conflict: please celebrate it. When conflict happens, two differing opinions or ideas are occurring at the same time. This is natural in any friendship and is a doorway to a deeper relationship. When my friend called me a female body part, he knew he was out of line. He apologized. I asked for some space to process his apology and to let myself emotionally regroup. I forgave him, and we became even better friends because of it.

*You*tilization

Sometimes, the best thing you can do to learn how to handle something well is to watch someone handle it badly. That's what I want you to do. Go to YouTube and watch at least one video of how Zach Galifianakis and his guests handle conflict in his show Between Two Ferns.

Wanna go even deeper?

Take some time to journal about your personal tendencies around conflict. Are you too quick to apologize and accept responsibility or are you always the person that's right? Share your observations with a therapist or close friend.

Keeping Friends: Jealousy and Envy

My daughter has a boyfriend. He's a great guy! He's smart, handsome, and seems to care a lot about the same things my daughter cares about. He also drives a really sweet truck and owns a gorgeous 2009, dark gray, Pontiac G8 with an upgraded, after-market cam shaft and upgraded long tube headers in the exhaust system (I think this makes it louder, but who knows). It is sa-weeeet! And ... his family has a cabin on a lake that she goes to every weekend. Other than being abnormally good looking, I've got none of those things. Enter ... jealousy.

Jealousy and envy are two unfortunate emotions we have to deal with as human beings. The problem is that they can get in the way of really great friendships. I described the situation with my daughter because it will help me better explain these two very similar terms. I've found that once these things are clearly defined and I've slapped a label on them, handling them is a lot easier. Name it, then solve it. I'm addressing jealousy and envy together because often I find myself using them interchangeably. But, I think there's a better way. What if we defined them differently? What if we made a distinction between the two? I think it could help! Let's give it a shot.

Jealousy is an emotion that occurs when you have something and there's a threat or fear of it being lost or taken away. It almost always happens between three people. I have a daughter, for example, that I love and cherish deeply. She is *my* daughter. Now, she has a boyfriend who is "threatening" to take her away from me through their deepening relationship. The jealousy I feel is a very natural response, but is it rational? Kind of. I know I'm not losing my relationship with her if she decides to marry this guy, but it will be different. I don't know about you, but I don't enjoy "different."

Envy is what you feel when someone has something you don't have but really want and the desire for it consumes you. It's hyper-admiration, self-pity, and bitterness rolled up into one very ugly mess. Envy typically happens between two people. Let's assume, for example, that my daughter's boyfriend's Pontiac G8 is a better car than my four-cylinder Ford Focus (big leap, I know, but you can do it). I'm already jealous of this guy because he has my daughter, but the fact that he has a sa-weeeeet car and he's not even forty yet just doesn't seem fair. I should have sa-weeeeet car. In fact, my opinion of this dude just dropped because I am so envious of him. Ok, so the envy stuff is made up. He does have a really sa-weeeet car, but I am quite smitten with my Ford Focus. Now that that's out of the way, let's dive a little deeper.

Once I've identified what the emotions are that I am dealing with (labeling them), I can begin to do healthy things with them (solving things). Jealousy isn't bad by itself, but what you do with it can be. When a person thinks their loved one is cheating on them, jealousy has been known to lead to a lot of actions that land people in jail. I would argue that envy isn't healthy in any form. If I envy someone because they've got a really cool car, this will not only affect my opinion of that person, but it also distracts me from being thankful for the blessings I *do* have in my life.

Like I said before, jealousy doesn't have to be all bad. It can direct you to change behavior and protect a relationship you may have been neglecting. A key component of jealousy is fear which can be a very healthy and even life-saving emotion. Envy is destructive without exception. Envy is fueled by bitterness and void of gratitude which is a very isolating situation to be in. It creates emotional barriers between us and other people when we constantly compare ourselves to them. It's like taking poison and expecting the other person to die.

Avoiding envy is easier said than done, but here are a couple ideas to get you started.

First, pay attention to when you're comparing yourself to others. It is so easy to fall into the comparison game. We can start to become envious and not even know it's happening. So when you find yourself doing the: "They have, they can, they are … I don't, I can't, I'm not" trap, I hope you remember this warning. Envy kills relationships. And then journal and talk to a friend or therapist about it. You're not alone. Envy may not be good, but it is normal.

Another solution to envy is to take it head on! Celebrate the success. Wait. What? Yes … you celebrate their great ... whatever. When someone you love gets something great or accomplishes something they've been working toward, it more than likely has been a journey for them. You may start to feel envious, but you can snub your nose at envy by being part of their celebration. Acknowledge what it has taken for your friend to get whatever they were working toward. You don't have to be dishonest and say you're happy for them if you're not, but the sooner you kick envy's butt, the sooner you *can* and *will* be happy for them. Happiness is often the result of good decisions followed by healthy actions.

The absolute nemesis of envy, which I've hinted to before, is gratitude. Take a look around. What do you have? What do you see around you that is beautiful and awesome? Focus on these things! Life will be so much sweeter if we all would.

What does all of this have to do with you, and what do you do about it? These two emotions, like many others, are difficult for people who struggle with a mental illness because it can be hard for us to deal with the influx of even one more emotional storm with a clear head. But when we're bound up in an emotional storm, it's our logical thoughts that will often help us get to where we need to be. This logical thought is referred to as using your *wisemind* in Dialectical Behavior Therapy (DBT).

When we face our emotional struggles head on, we see them for what they really are: the reflections of our brokenness. Do you want to be happy for your loved ones when they succeed? Would you like them to celebrate and be excited when you succeed? We can't make ourselves feel a certain way, but we can pave the way for the emotions we want to feel through conscious decisions that lead to action. Through our carefully chosen actions, we allow the natural course of events to lead toward a positive outcome. Remember that journal thing? I've found that when I am reluctant to admit a struggle to another person, or even out loud to myself, a journal is a wonderful and safe place to go. I write out as honestly as I can what my struggle is regardless of how petty it feels or how embarrassed I am to admit it. It doesn't even have to be legible (see journaling rules chapter for more info), just get it down on paper.

So figure out what you feel. Label it. Then stare that emotion straight in the eye. Revolt. Rebel. Love those whom you envy. Celebrate with them and watch your quality- of-life soar.

*You*tilization

Is there anyone in your life you are envious of? Your *You*tilization challenge is to write a letter or call someone to congratulate or celebrate their good fortune, then watch the envy melt away.

Wanna go even deeper?

Go to your journal and write about an experience you witnessed (of either you or someone you know) where jealousy or envy caused big problems. Were there any lessons learned? Have you ever experienced a time when jealousy brought about a positive outcome ... where the fear of losing something caused you to take action to cherish or value something more?

Keeping Friends: Boundaries

When you care about something, you create boundaries around it. Take your health for example. When you care for your body and show concern about your overall health, you set boundaries. What does that look like? You go to the gym, eat more of certain foods, and less or none of others. Creating boundaries isn't as much about setting limitations on something as it is about protecting and cherishing it.

Consider your favorite brand of chocolate milk. You would never take that delicious Tru Moo, uncap it, then pour it onto the counter. That would be ridiculous. No. Instead you grab a glass, place it on the counter and pour the delightfully delicious drink into it. The glass is a boundary mechanism. It contains the chocolate milk so that it can be enjoyed. How does this play out in our friendships?

Most people, in my experience, don't sit down with their friends and read out a list of things they will and won't do, or things they do and don't like. No, we learn these things about each other as we develop our relationships together. So, what does it look like to pour our friendships into a glass? I have a friend that goes to bed at nine p.m. every night. I don't get to bed until around midnight, and most of my messages with my friends happen between nine and midnight because that works for them. But I know my friend Mike is in bed at nine p.m., and so I try to communicate with him before that. This is something that's important to him. If he wouldn't have told me about this, and I just kept messaging or calling past nine, this would put a strain on our relationship. Likewise, he knows that I don't drink alcohol, (have you caught on yet that I prefer chocolate milk?) so he doesn't waste precious time trying to get me to drink. When he invites me over, he usually has a half gallon of the local brown cow brew on hand. Spelling out personal boundaries to the ones we love helps us connect better and leaves little room for guesswork or assumptions. Life is already too much of a guessing game. Setting and communicating boundaries is something you can do to make it easier on your friends and yourself.

What happens to a friendship when those boundaries are not clear? Remember that chocolate yumminess that gets all over the counter because you chose not to pour it into a glass? Yep ... that's your friendship. A mess. Tough to clean up. Spread thin. Not very enjoyable. Not to mention, it can get all over other things like your clothes, other food, and clean dishes on the counter. When one part of our lives get messy, it rarely ever stays contained. If you don't set boundaries, it will inevitably affect other areas of your life. Fortunately for you, it works both ways.

When you're drinking that delicious chocolate milk, perfectly held within the boundary created by the glass, it tastes so good going down. When you and your friends understand each others' boundaries, it feels so great and just adds to the joy of life. That mutual understanding and respect is so delicious, isn't it?

Let's talk specifics. What kind of boundaries should we think about setting?

- **Behaviors:** My wife and I have an arrangement that I mentioned earlier in the book. I am very uncomfortable with a lot that happens during a wedding reception so before all those shenanigans begin, I head to the car and read a book or find something else to do. I understand that there are times, especially within a marriage, that you may need to do what isn't necessarily comfortable. But that's why you talk it out with your friend. If something is extremely uncomfortable and doesn't require your attention or attendance, and if you and your friend agree on it, then avoidance isn't such a bad idea.

- **Safety:** Never compromise on safety. Whether you're dared by a friend to do something dangerous or you're in a physical, emotional, or verbally abusive relationship, never compromise your safety.

- **Time:** One of the things that bothers me is when a friend constantly shows up late when we are hanging out. If it's just once or twice, no big deal. But if it's their habit, then it really starts to get under my skin. If we have a set time to hang out, I feel validated when my friend shows up on time and feel that they don't want to be there if they show up late. This happens with one of my friends who's late every time we hang out. It's disappointing because I seldom have time to hang out with friends. Respect your friend's time, please. And if you have a friend who is constantly late, talk to them. Figure out what is going on and let them know how it makes you feel. You can save yourself a ton of heartache by putting yourself out there like this.

• **Reciprocation:** This is an interesting boundary concept that I have come to value as I get older. It's the reciprocation boundary. By reciprocation, I mean the back and forth, give and take nature of friendship. It's the equality and balance we have among friends. Have you ever had a friend that constantly asks for stuff, but rarely has anything to offer? That gets old, right? But what about that friend who never asks for anything? That's a problem too, isn't it? I constantly remind my friends that I want to help them. It sets my heart on fire. Do you have a friend that's always willing to listen to your problems, but doesn't really open up about theirs? That's a problem, right? Because, how can you relate to that? It's happened to me. It feels like they are holding back because they don't fully trust you. You can't have a relationship if you can't relate. And you can't relate to someone who won't ask for help or share their problems with you.

- **Energy:** Here is something that I need to pay more attention to! How do you feel when you are around your friend? Do you come away from your time together feeling energized or drained? This isn't being selfish or shallow, but I've got to be honest, it kind of feels like it is. I can't tell you how often I've punished myself by hanging out with really, really great people who leave me feeling empty and lonelier inside than if I had just stayed home by myself. Please don't do that to yourself. I understand that not every hang-out session will be energizing, but you should pay attention to how you feel. Most of the time, at least, you should leave with your heart feeling full and your mind/body energized.

- **Personal support:** Do you feel that you can be honest with your friend? Can you give your honest opinion to this person, have them accept it, and respect it without dismissing you? Are you always expected to agree with them? I know that it can be super awkward to disagree with a friend, but it doesn't have to be something that will tear the relationship apart. Whether it's a disagreement about the best band, best food, a political, or social issue, you don't have to agree on everything. And ... you won't, but that's a good thing. Are you both able and willing to accept each other despite your differences? If all I drank was chocolate milk 24/7, I would die from a chocolate milk overdose, and, even worse, I'd end up being sick of it. Really. It's not that healthy. I drink water, sweet tea, and another big favorite, smoothies. Diversity in all things breeds excitement. Embrace those who think differently than you. Don't hang out with people who won't accept you for you.

What do you do if someone compromises one of your boundaries? First, ask your friend if they knew the boundary even existed. If they didn't, then let them know. Most often, situations like these are misunderstandings. If they did know about the boundary, then just talk to them about it. It may be super awkward, but these types of conversations are what lifelong friendships are built on.

*You*tilization

Think about some of the boundaries you and your friends already have? What are they? Record them in your journal and why they're there.

Wanna go even deeper?

Take some time to journal about your personal tendencies around conflict. Are you too quick to apologize and accept responsibility, or are you always the person that's right? Share your observations with a therapist or close friend.

Keeping Friends: Accountability

One of the most amazing gifts that friendship can give us is the ability to help keep our integrity and achieve goals. Is there an area in your life that you'd like to improve? Stuff you'd like to do? Do your friends know what they are? Because ... they should. And if they know, are they helping you achieve those goals? Because ... I bet they'd want to!

A few years back, I wanted to build a seventeen-foot-tall beer bottle constructed out of PVC and panhandler-style cardboard signs for an international art competition. The project's name was Missing People. I needed a lot of support. People plan for these types of things for years. I put a team together and began planning just six months before the competition started. But I was inspired, and so me and a rag-tag group of amazing people dove headfirst into this crazy project. I desperately needed accountability. I needed someone to remind me the reason why I was doing this and that I was not alone. Along with my team, several friends helped hold me accountable, encouraging me to keep pushing forward, often on a daily basis.

What is accountability? Well, let's start with the word "account." In Joe-terms, it means to measure against expectations. Then "ability" means, in Joe-terms, well ... ability. Thus, accountability is an agreement between x number of people to encourage someone to achieve a specific expectation. What makes or breaks accountability is all a matter of execution. As a twenty-something man, I thought accountability was about power and authority. That intimidation and consequences were how you helped people do what they wanted to get done. That type of accountability is unsustainable. Why? Because that kind of relationship is unsustainable. Relationships driven by fear and condemnation are not healthy, and thereby not sustainable.

A combination lock has several dials or numbers that need to be positioned in a specific way for it to be opened. If you want to use accountability to help open up your potential, here's the combination: remind, encourage, relate, be vulnerable, and be honest. The first three points of this combo relate specifically to the friend giving the support. The last two points are important for both people. One of the best ways to help someone get something done, which is the whole reason for accountability, is to remind them why they're doing it. I was building a humongous beer bottle, for example, because I wanted to remind everyone who saw it to love a certain group of people in their lives.

It's encouraging when a person has a goal and they know that it's important to more than just themselves. So having friends rooting for you and understanding the purpose of the goal is extremely helpful. Most goals have physical or emotional obstacles to overcome, so when the process gets hard, it's so important to have people standing in your corner.

Relating is also crucial because it's so helpful when someone strives to understand the hard work that's going into the goal. No one else can really completely understand as well as the person in the trenches, but their willingness to try makes a world of difference.

Whenever someone asks a friend for help, there's always the potential for problems. When we acknowledge our need for help, we are simultaneously admitting our limitations. Sharing our weaknesses and limitations are the building blocks of trust. When I was working on the Missing People project, I needed a lot of money, a space to build, and some specific supplies. It was an expression of vulnerability to go to my friends and ask for help. An accountability partner is very beneficial when they are vulnerable and admit to their own weaknesses as a way to relate and encourage the other person.

Last, but certainly not least, accountability depends heavily on honesty. The accountability partner needs to be honest about how they perceive the friend's actions lining up with the initial goals. The friend needs to openly communicate the goal's progress to their partner in order to get helpful feedback.

Here are some simple steps for starting an accountability relationship. The first thing, which may seem uber-obvious, is to have something specific you want to do. That's your goal. Once you've got that decided, make a list of the people who truly care about you, who'd care about what you're trying to do, and are fairly decent communicators. Then, sit down with them and explain what you want to do and why. Lastly, set a start and end date. Decide when you want the accountability relationship to begin and end. It's not ok to keep these things open ended. It can create a lot of awkwardness in the relationship—and relationships are already awkward enough. So do yourself a favor, set the dates.

If you're asked to be someone's accountability partner, that's a pretty big deal. Make sure you think long and hard about it before you make your decision. Do you completely understand what they're asking you to do? Are you capable of following through? If you're the one doing the asking, give your friend a while to think it over. This is one of the most rewarding things friends can do for each other. *Every time* I've had one these relationships, I've accomplished some incredible stuff. I know you will, too.

*You*tilization

Do you have a goal? Even a tiny one? Tell someone about it. Ask a friend to be your accountability partner. Once you've brought an accountability partner into the scenario, the accomplishment goes beyond just one person. It becomes the achievement of a team. When the goal is completed, celebrate your accomplishment with that friend.

Wanna go even deeper?

Talk to your friend and ask them about their goals. Then offer your services as an accountability partner. This will help you practice what you've learned or been inspired to do and, more importantly, it will be a wonderful thing for you to do for your friend.

Keeping Friends: Helping Friends in Crisis

"This is a story about four people named Everybody, Somebody, Anybody, and Nobody. One day there was a very sad and lonely person that just needed Somebody to care. So, Everybody was asked to help. Everybody was sure Somebody would do it. Anybody could have done it, but Nobody did it. Somebody got angry about that, because it was Everybody's job. Everybody thought Anybody could do it but Nobody realized that Everybody wouldn't do it. The friend ended up dying alone in their depression. Everybody blamed Somebody when Nobody did what Anybody could have done."

Author Unknown

This chapter contains potential emotional triggers due to the subject matter: Suicide.

It was the last day I'd get to see my best friend. I was boiling with anger, bitten by confusion, and drowning in waves of grief. The church was packed. Every seat, every spot to stand was layered with bewildered friends and family. I was lumbering around trying to find somewhere I fit in. That's when my friend Jacobi texted to see if there was anything I needed. Isn't it crazy how huge the simplest acts of kindness can feel? Thirty minutes before the ceremony, she was dragging her kids around the city to find me a sandwich and some sweet tea.

His name was Nathan Beals. We first met at a leadership retreat in 2013. We hit it off right away! We loved each other like brothers. In fact, despite our differences—which were many—he always introduced me as his long-lost twin brother from another mother. Our relationship went from zero to sixty when, a few months after we met, I landed in the same psychiatric hospital he'd just been released from.

There's something I need you to understand about this guy. He was a giant, both literally and figuratively. This guy, all six-feet seven-inches and four-hundred pounds of him, was a force to be reckoned with. He'd been a husband, adopted father of eight, pastor, friend to hundreds, and staunch advocate for mental health. This dear friend of mine, who fought so aggressively and passionately for the broken hearts of so many people, gave up hope and the exhausting battle with his illness, on January 24th, 2018. A lot had happened to him that year before his death. He'd lost his marriage, abandoned his kids, quit his job as a pastor, and fell off the social radar of most of the people who had loved him. He was a friend living in crisis.

What can you do for someone you care so very much about when they are in such an obvious emotional tailspin? One of the things Nathan was known for was just showing up. If he knew you were having a bad day, there'd be a knock at your door and a huge, smiling,

Black man standing there, excited to remind you that you were loved. I don't think there is a perfect answer to the question of what to do when a friend is in crisis, but I think Nathan gave us all a clue: Just do something. When he was struggling, I kept reminding myself to just. do. something. I'd call, text, or hang out whenever both of us were available. He didn't make it easy, though. He insulted me. Ignored me. But I just kept showing up. Why? Because that's what friends do.

Wanna know what I think is royally messed up? Who's the most qualified person to prepare friends for your crisis?

You are.
You and only you.

Sure, friends can show up, but beyond that, helping is a crapshoot … unless you prepare them. Who's better equipped than you to help your friends love you better? Yeah, it sucks that you have to do the legwork to help others around you know how to love and support you when you're hurting. And it's not something you want to wait to do until you're in a crisis. But, since you're reading this, it's not something you have to figure out alone.

This idea, preparing your friends and yourself for emotional crises, is called "coping-ahead." Shortly after Nathan passed away, I had to go to the hospital for a lung biopsy. The doctors found a large mass on my left lung and feared it was cancer. Just before the procedure, I sent a message to my closest friends, giving them a heads up about what was going on and how they could love me depending on the outcome. I was scared, and I needed a lot of support. You and I have both experienced how difficult it can be for someone on the outside of an emotional struggle to know how to help. That's why coping-ahead is so great! It gives the people who care about you the permission and instruction to know how to help. What a great gift!

So, that spot on my lung ended up being something called organized pneumonia. The treatment for this rare condition lasted two years, until the mass dissipated. And my amazing friends were there for me through it all.

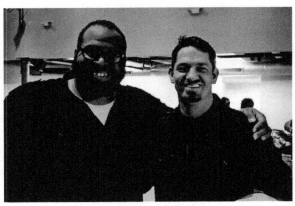

Me and my friend, Nathan.

*You*tilization

Make a list in your journal of the things that would be helpful for your friends to know and do for you when you find yourself in an emotional crisis. At the same time, it doesn't do any good for you to keep this list to yourself. Share this idea and your list with a few close friends.

Wanna go even deeper?

Call one of your good friends and ask for a few ideas that would help them when they're struggling. Right this next to your list in your journal. This is also something you'll want to record in your Friend Files, which I'm going to tell you about in a little bit.

INTENTIONAL BEST FRIENDS

A little background

In 2002, I had very few boundaries and a lot going on. Whenever a friend needed anything, I felt an unhealthy amount of responsibility to do something about it, and I usually did. Considering the fact that, at the time, I had a wife and two young children, worked full-time, and volunteered several hours a week at my church, I was living a very imbalanced life. I was destined for a breakdown. I needed a change. Then I *had* that breakdown. I needed some boundaries. Intentional Best Friends (IBF) became that boundary.

When Thanksgiving in 2003 rolled around, I came up with the idea to make a list of the top ten people I was thankful for that year. We'd had quite a bit happen in our family, and I had a lot to be grateful for. So I made the list and sent each person a letter, and it felt great to acknowledge these people who helped carry my family through the year. In the letter, I let them know what they did that had meant so much to our family and that they were part of an exclusive group.

After doing this for a few years, I realized that these people were more than just people I was thankful for … the list was mostly made up of people I considered to be my best friends. A few of them were therapists that

218

helped my son and wife with some specific things going on in their lives at the time, but the majority of them were my closest friends. So I decided I needed to make a change. This change would forever alter how I did friendship. I decided to organize a core group of friends that would help me establish healthy boundaries. That's when I created IBF.

When IBF started, I called it Ten Friends because I felt challenged to see if I could come up with a list of ten people. I felt the need to stretch myself. It wasn't easy at first. I've always wrestled with thoughts of worthlessness and that I was destined to be alone. I decided there needed to be zero expectations from these people. Then I chose the ten people I cared about and admired the most and wrote them a letter. This was purely an investment in and commitment to them. In my mind, keeping the commitment one-sided reduced the risk of rejection and disappointment. I should have known better, but you don't know what you don't know, and you've got to start somewhere.

*You*tilization

I want to get you thinking about making a personal and intentional investment in the people that matter most to you, so grab your journal and make a list of all your friends. These are the people you enjoy talking to at church, school, and work. They don't have to be your best friend. Just someone you'd consider a friend. Keep this list, we will use it later.

Wanna go even deeper?

After you've made your list of friends, make another list of people you admire most. Only people you have access to. People you'd be able to get in touch with because you know their address, phone number, email, etc. Is there an overlap between the two lists? Circle the names that are on both.

IBF: Mindfulness

Near the beginning of the book, I shared a few traumatizing situations I experienced while I was at an inpatient psychiatric facility in West Michigan. It was terrifying and borderline ridiculous. This has had a profound impact on how I view inpatient psychiatric facilities. I never wanted to go to one ever again! But ... I ended up needing too, and I was absolutely terrified. The next time I went to a psychiatric hospital, it was a completely different experience, thank God. A lot had changed in the mental health world from 2002 to 2013. Medication for mental illness was still an important *part* of the treatment plan, but only one part. At the time, I'd been seeing a counselor that taught DBT. Taught?! What a fantastic concept for counselors and therapists. This was the program I'd needed my entire life. For me, it was kind of like the idiot's guide to common sense *and* a how-to program for dealing with life's normal ups and downs, all rolled up into one neat little package. I don't know anyone that enjoys dealing with conflict, anxiety, distress, and tragedy, but DBT taught me how to manage difficult situations like these in a way that wouldn't leave me catatonic.

One of the cornerstone tools of DBT is something called "mindfulness." Mindfulness is the idea that a person is better off emotionally when they're thinking about what they are doing while and where they're doing it. One aspect of mindfulness that I struggle with the most is paying attention to what I'm thinking about. On the surface this sounds easy, right? But, one of the biggest traps I find myself falling into is trying to do and think too much all at once because I've learned that this is somehow better and more productive. Learning mindfulness has taught me to slow down. To simplify. To ... relax.

There's probably been many times throughout your life when you felt like some kind of light switch went on in your head. You've learned or experienced something that changed your life. Mindfulness was that for me. A big, frigging light switch. I was doing and thinking way too much!

"But I thought God wasn't supposed to give me more than I could handle." Isn't that what the Bible says? I mean, I saw all these "needs" that needed to get done. Even now I as I write this, I struggle with wanting to think and do too much. But I now realize that just because I see a problem, doesn't mean I am solely responsible for solving it (more on that a little later). Problems never end, right? And if you spend time following the cause and effect of them, they only get bigger. The mental and emotional rabbit holes you'll find yourself going down will seem endless. The guilt. The ambition. The pride. It's overwhelming.

So, what does this have to do with friendship? And what is an "Intentional Best Friend (IBF)?" I'm getting there. But first I want you to understand the process I've gone through to get me to where I am. I want you to understand one of the biggest players that has led to how I "do friendship." I can't go back to living in the chaos I found myself a decade ago, and mindfulness has played a key role in developing one of my strongest allies in this struggle: my friends.

*You*tilization

Grab a blanket and a book or some music and go find a quiet park or grassy knoll. Go lay down. Read your book. Listen to your music. But practice being all there. Run your hand lightly over the grass next to you. Let it tickle your arms. Just. Be. All. There.

Wanna go even deeper?

While you're laying down, take few minutes to engage the five senses. What do you see, hear, taste, feel, and smell? Before you leave your little spot, journal about your experience. Answer this question: What stood out to me while I was laying there? What got my attention?

IBF: Getting Started

The Nuts and Bolts

Intentional Best Friendship is a tight-knit community of best friends that I choose every Thanksgiving. It's an exclusive group of people that I devote myself to for the next 365 days. Many people stay on the list year after year. But, as with most friendships, there is an ebb and flow. People come and go from the list. I'll get more into this later.

Here are a few of the big "why's" for this list:

- **It takes away your excuse for self-pity.** When self-pity sets in and you feel like you're all alone in this world, you know who your closest friends are. You've got a list and it's written down.

- **It simplifies your commitment issues.** Sometimes I don't know where to stop when it comes to helping someone in need, and, at other times, I feel like I don't do enough. IBF gives you boundaries. You're going to learn to give yourself the freedom to reject the guilt that comes with telling your friends "no" when they ask for something. You're also going to learn that you can't always say "yes" to your IBF. But this list gives you emotional boundaries that you'll find easy to function within. In a case where you have two people who need your help, if one of those people is an IBF, your decision is easy. Of course things like severity of need, time, opportunity, and resources all play a part in making that decision, but all things being equal ... you will side with your IBF.

- **You know who to ask for help.** If you ever find yourself needing help, you know where to turn. You can ask one of your IBFs. It's also great to let them know that if they ever need help, you want them to come to you. These are the people you have learned you can count on!

- **They understand your struggle.** Your IBFs are the people you'll cope-ahead with and teach the Mental Health Scale to. And, when you're struggling in the negative zone, they will help you move in the right direction. They also know who to contact when you're getting close to, or are at, your crisis number.

*You*tilization is key when it comes to introducing IBFs into your life. I started with the number ten. But it can be any number you want or need. In fact, my list has been as large as twelve and as small as three. It really just depends on the year and what's happening in your life at the time (this year there just so happens to be a pandemic ... lucky us!). The key is to make the list, whatever number it may be, and then to follow through with next steps.

A small group of friends, my wife, and I used to go to a neighborhood in our city that we felt could use some encouragement. We'd bring bags of bagels, walk around to all the different apartments, and give them away. We'd also spend time talking about life and asking if there was anything we could pray about with them. We weren't trying to be pushy, just trying to be present. Every once in a while, a few people would hear about what we were doing and would come along and help. One of those people, a young lady, was astonished by how much we knew about the community and about the individual families within that community. She asked me how we could possibly know so much. "When you care, you know." Isn't that the truth? When you care about someone, you know about them and are excited to learn more. The same goes with an IBF. You know them and will love getting to know them more and more every day.

The process begins with authenticity. Maybe you think this sounds like a piece of cake. I assure you, it's harder than it sounds. We spend too much time looking at people that are "better than us." Admiring them, trying to copy their behaviors. It's no wonder we forget who we are. Don't believe the lie, that there is something wrong with you—at least not anything more wrong than the next person. Everyone goes through seasons of life where they're trying to be like someone else. The truth is, we'd like ourselves a whole lot more if we'd learn to see and accept the beauty of our own uniqueness. Be authentic. Allow yourself to like the things you like, even if you're the only one on the planet that does. It takes a lot of time and effort to shed the person you were pretending to be because it took a lot of time and effort to become the person you never were. But it's totally worth it. Learning to be honest with and about yourself will be a huge first step toward learning to be honest with and about your friendships.

So, let's start to figure out your IBFs.

Step 1: Make a list of all your friends, acquaintances, and people you'd like to have as one of your IBFs.

This first step is a pretty straightforward process. If you did your *You*tilization activity at the end of the Nailing It chapter, you're all set! Otherwise, grab your journal and write the names of every friend, acquaintance, or potential friend you have. One other thing before you start writing: refer back to the Mental Health Scale. Where are you at on the scale right now? If you're anywhere near your crisis number, wait until you're closer to zero or, better yet, at a positive number to do this. You'll find it nearly impossible to come up of a good list if you're not doing even close to emotionally well.

Step 2: Make a list of what's important to you.

This second step can be a little intimidating, but don't worry, I'm here to help. You've already read about what's important to me in the chapters about journaling: God, Health, Family, and Myself. Of course, a lot falls under these categories, but those pretty much sum it up. What are the characteristics of a friend that are important to you? There are the basics: honesty, trustworthiness, fun, and shared interests (especially chocolate milk). Maybe you'd add: godly character, wisdom, business savvy, availability, sincerity, tenderness, intentionality, proximity, and good looks. The list could go on forever. Have you ever considered a person's size, race, how much money they make, or how old they are? No, not as a means of excluding people. What I'm asking is, do you have friends that look different than you, live in a different neighborhood, or come from a different era. No matter who you are, I think it's important to invite people into our lives that are different from us. Take a look at the list of friends you wrote down. Do they all look like you? Do they all make about the same amount of money as you do? How old are they? Stretch yourself. Who else can you add to that list that may be just a little bit different?

My mom and dad typically eat at one of two restaurants near Detroit when they go out: Baldos, an Italian pizza place, and Pete's Place, which serves just about anything considered to be normal American food. That's what I ate growing up. We ate the same meals because it's what we knew. It's what we were comfortable with. Then ... I met my wife. Yo, the first time she cooked for me, she put fungus in my spaghetti sauce! I'd never had mushrooms before. But I was trying to impress her, so I chewed them, and then eventually allowed them to travel down my esophagus. Now? I love fungus. I can't get enough of it! There are so many awesome foods I never would have tried had I not opened myself up to something different.

I am a 6'4", white, thin, middle class, male. If I only hung out with people who are just like me, I'd be missing out on a lot of great experiences. Everyone has a tendency to associate with people who are just like them. It happens on social media all the time. People are drawn toward other people that look and think like they do. Why? Because it's comfortable. It's familiar. It reinforces beliefs and ideas we already hold to be true and sidelines our fears and insecurities. These people aren't bad, but they only reinforce the narrative the person friending them has already established in their mind. I'm not saying you need to have best friends that are fatter or thinner than you, richer or poorer. What I do want you to do is to look at the friends you have. Is there any group left out? Then ask why that group is not represented. That's all I want. You may find out things about yourself and the world around you when you open up your friendships and perspective to a wider variety of people and ideas.

One of the things I consider quite seriously when deciding on an IBF is whether or not this relationship will be one-sided. I mentioned earlier that when I first started this process, I had no expectations from these friends. That's changed. Why? Consider the word *relationship*. The root word of relationship is relate. If we can't have that, if we can't be equitable toward one another, if we can't relate, then this friend-*ship's* not going to float, and there is no us. It's quite normal for a friendship to be emotionally one-sided during a crisis or difficult season. It's equally normal for friendships to go through seasons of physical or emotional distance. But on the whole, there should be a give and take balance among friends.

Step 3. Decide on the number.

Please don't spend too much time on this step. In fact, if you think about it for longer than five minutes, you're trying too hard. Here's what I want you to do. Think about all the people you have in your life that you'd consider best friends. I think most of us have a small number—maybe one to three people. I'd like for you, if your number is below five, to come up with a number that is at least double that. If your number is greater than five, you should probably keep it where it is. If it's greater than ten, you might want to trim it down. These are the friends who will receive gifts from you on their birthdays. They are the ones who, when they ask for prayer, you will actually pray for. Your limitations are really just time, money, and level of creativity: Do you have the time to spend with each person individually? If so, do you have financial limits that may become an obstacle if you decided to buy gifts for them on their birthdays or Christmas. Will you have time and the emotional fortitude to pray for these friends? Maybe write those prayers out? These are just a few things that you might want to consider. Think about what you want to do and multiply that by the number of close friends you'll have. I know when my number was twelve, it was a bit overwhelming. I felt like I wasn't able to invest in each friend like I really wanted to. Challenge yourself to have a number that might stretch who you are without breaking your emotional bank.

Write that number here: _____

Step 4. Select your Intentional Best Friends

This is where the rubber meets the road. You've listed your friends, decided what things are important to you, and also figured out how many friends are manageable. Now all you need to determine is the who. But you can do it! Don't just think about what you will receive in the next year from these people, but also what you have to offer them. It's about symbiosis. There is a beautiful give and take to these relationships. What will this person contribute to your life? What can you contribute to theirs? Maybe you don't have an answer for that. That's ok! You just really admire the person and don't know why. That's fine. I say, go for it. Just be mindful as you are interacting with your friends through the year, to avoid the one-sidedness that can happen. Maybe you don't see how your friendship benefits the other person. That's not a reason not to try! Talk to them about it. Tell them you value equality and want to be as big a blessing to them as you know they will be to you. As you discuss this together, I have no doubt your eyes will be opened to some of your unique abilities and gifts, and it'll deepen your bond with your friend.

So, you've got your list.
Now pick a launch date that's important to you.
Write down the date that you've chosen:

_____

What's next? Here are a couple things you can do with your list.

Keep it a secret

An IBF is a really cool way to develop the meaningful friendships and personal support essential for improving mental health. With that said, one option to consider when doing this is to keep it a secret. Just create your list, and on day one, start doing the intentional thing. You don't announce it to anyone. There's no showy invitation. You just make the list, and then commit to developing and cherishing these relationships for the next 365 days.

Why in the world would you want to keep this idea a secret? Well, for starters, most friendships don't last forever. Even the best of friends come and go. Do you see how this might create some extra stress in your life down the road? It's important to remember that your IBF list is not just a group of friends, but an exclusive collection of your closest friends. And as life happens, circumstances change, and people move on, your list will change. People grow apart or find new friends. Some people will be an IBF one year but not the next. This happens for lots of reasons. In the fifteen-plus years I've been doing this, I've only had one instance when the list I had from one year was the same exact list for the following year. Having people coming and going from this list can add a bit of stress to your life. How? Let's say your friend Bill has been one of your IBFs for the last five years, but this year you two have been a little distant and you can sense a shift in the depth of your friendship. You're still friends and care deeply for each other, but you're just not as close as you once were. You both have moved on and your IBF list should reflect that. If Bill has been on your list the last five years, and this is something he has been aware of, receiving some sort of notification of that fact, then he may wonder what happened this year. It is that *wondering* that can be difficult for the IBF, and the fear that you may hurt them. So when the big day rolls around, if you are making the list public, and Bill realizes he isn't chosen, it could get really awkward. Bill may even feel a little hurt. It's easy to avoid hard feelings and disappointing people when you have a special list of friends that is completely unknown to them. I liken it to a competition where I am the only person that knows it's a competition. That way, when the other person loses, they don't feel bad. And they ALWAYS lose.

Another advantage to keeping this idea a secret, is that you don't risk all of your other friends who are not on this exclusive list, making them feel like second class friends. This is not the intention of IBF, but it is understandable why someone would feel this way. The purpose of this list isn't to create different classes of friends, rather it is to create personal boundaries in your life to help with your mental health. Class systems say that one person is better or more deserving than another. IBFs say that one friend is more likely to get my attention, effort, and time than another friend for the purposes of creating a balanced life.

I am very outspoken about doing Intentional Best Friends because I think it is a really good idea, and I want people to know about it. It is my hope that when people see it openly modelled, they will be encouraged to think more intentionally about their friendships. I know this isn't for everyone, but for me, it has been a game changer! Have there been some hurt feelings? I honestly don't know. Probably? Life is full of disappointments though. Everyone that knows I do this knows why and that I struggle with mental illness. They know I constantly battle to do things that will help me live a fuller life, and at the same time, try to help people around me do the same. So you could save yourself the headache of explaining this to a bunch of people by just keeping it a secret.

Make it a BIG DEAL

I once attended a culinary class that my daughter enrolled me in as a birthday gift. One of the things I learned is that you eat with your eyes first. It's the idea that if the food is well presented and looks delicious, it will trigger a part of your brain that makes you even more excited about the meal, adding to the overall good feelings you have about the experience. This works with friendship, too.

I love to make a fairly big deal about the process. Every year at Thanksgiving, I get out crisp white sheets of stationary and matching envelopes. I open a package of brand-new Pilot G-2 pens, size .07, and get my wax sealing kit ready to go. When I let people know that they are on this unique list, I want them to know it is something I have thought long and hard about; I want them to experience something special … the feeling of being *chosen*.

I want them to realize that I have chosen to invest an entire year in them. It's not a complicated process. I write out a very personal letter using my best printing, taking the time to tell them what they mean to me and why I selected them. Then I invite them into this new relationship. I seal the envelope with wax and either mail it or make a special trip to their house Thanksgiving Day to give it to them.

It doesn't really matter what day you choose to do this, but it would be helpful if the day had some sort of special meaning for you. I chose Thanksgiving because IBF started as a list of the ten people I was most thankful for in my life. At the time, one of my children was dealing with some trauma and my wife was getting ready to undergo bariatric surgery. Despite the difficult circumstances, there was a whole lot I had to be thankful for and this was the way I chose to express it. You can choose Christmas and use your announcement as a recognition of the gifts that friends are in your life. New Year's Day could signify a new year and a new start. Use your birthday to celebrate who you are and who you want to be! Find the reason to do this whenever it feels right for you.

Having the talk

If you decide to make a big deal out of Intentional Best Friends, there is one more thing I want you to do. When you are ready to send out your letters and begin a new year of commitments, be considerate to the people who are not returning to the list. Don't just leave them hanging, wondering if they will or won't get a letter. It would go a long way toward saving yourself and the other person a lot of grief to let them know. Tell them what you've appreciated about their friendship and remind them that they are still your friend and you care for them. I always let my IBFs know that it is only a commitment for the next 365 days and may not continue past that point for any number of reasons. You can even ask them if and how they'd prefer to be told if they didn't make it the following year. The key here—and the heart behind this—is not to hurt anybody's feelings but about setting healthy boundaries for a healthier you.

*You*tilization

Follow the four steps for creating your IBF list. Even if it's not something you're sure you want to do, go through the steps. It's always good to think intentionally about your friendships.

Wanna go even deeper?

If this is something you're considering doing, think about what date or special occasion works best for you. Then, decide if you want your IBFs to be something your friends know about, or something you keep to yourself. Then do it.

IBF: Friend Files

I'm the kind of guy that watches a movie, and then daydreams about doing the cool stuff I see on the screen. I want to be the hero! As a kid, I wanted be Daniel LaRusso from Karate Kid, and Superman's Clark Kent. As an adult, I enjoy movies with secrets. I've even talked to my wife about putting a secret room in our house like Corrie ten Boom's (and many others) who did this during World War II to hide people from persecution and death. I write coded letters to friends, and there was one time that I wrote to them in "invisible ink." I swear I followed the Youtube directions to the tee, but most of the text didn't turn out, and the letters were ruined. I want to be a hero for the people who matter most to me and so … I've created files for each of my family members and closest friends. I've got their favorite foods, important dates, names of family members, personal habits, and Meyers Briggs Personality Types. I also include things that I learn about them when we hang out. One of those people is my friend, Jeff.

Jeff is one of those guys that's not easy to get to know at first. He's very quiet. He would much rather just sit and listen to you talk. But I was committed to finding a way into his life and he seemed committed to watching me try. This guy is a deeply passionate and surprisingly emotional person. It takes him a while to trust others with his deeper self … unless you're me, apparently. It took all of ninety seconds to dig into his life and find out what made this guy tick. I think he's just looking for the right people to ask the right questions. How did it happen? Well, for starters, for one of our very first deep conversations, I dragged him into my somewhat cluttered bedroom—which my wife thought was a really weird thing to do. It seemed to make complete sense to me. We needed privacy. At the same time, I was in the process of learning how to be a little less reserved. I think my vulnerability created experiences of trust so that he became willing to open up to me. He has one of the bravest personalities I know. And, I've got a feeling, that this guy is going to be a friend for a long time. It's just the way he is. There is a mutual respect and love for each other because we are committed to being authentically us.

My friend Mike is great. We are always talking about deep stuff and encouraging each other toward one goal or another. But sometimes we disagree. I don't like it. It's not comfortable to disagree with someone you love. Not because I think he is wrong, but rather, I'm bothered because I don't want the disagreements to come between us. I want it to make us closer. How does that work? Well, for starters, it's important to recognize our own arrogance. The sooner we are able to identify that we don't hold all the keys to the doorway of truth, the better. I'm not saying that we should ever abandon what we believe to be true, but that we hold what we believe to be true in an open palm. That we be willing to confirm it or give up our stance, in time, in light of the evidence. Mike and I still don't agree about everything, but I think this makes us better friends than if we did, or pretended to.

I have this beautiful friend. Her name is Jacobi. She's married to my buddy, Jeff. During a conversation with her a while back, she said she didn't know what to do for her friends when they're hurting or sick. This goes back to something I mentioned before, and especially applies to people with a mental health condition. Take the time to communicate with your friends. Talk to them about what would help you when you're struggling. This is all part of the coping-ahead strategy. So I wrote down what Jacobi told me in her friend file. Knowing this about Jacobi has been very helpful for the both of us. On my forty-first birthday, while I was in the hospital recovering from a lung biopsy surgery gone wrong, I felt a sense of duty and empowerment and boldly asked her to bring me my favorite brand of chocolate moo brew. She did, and it was perfect … for both of us. One more note about coping-ahead. Ask your friends what would be helpful if they ever find themselves in an emotional storm. Then record it in their friend file for a rainy day. This is you coping-ahead for them.

I mentioned before that I keep track of my friends Meyers Briggs results. The Meyers Briggs Type Indicator is a personality test that I use to get to know my friends' preferences and worldview a little bit better. I just sent them a link to the free version and asked them to take it (www.16personalities.com). If they agreed with the result, they emailed it back to me. This Meyers Briggs thing, just like most things in life, isn't one-hundred percent foolproof, but chances are, you're going to learn something to help you be a better friend. And more than likely, you'll find deeper clues as to what makes your friends tick. Jacobi is a really good example of this. Her Meyers Briggs personality is ESFJ.

> "ESFJs are consistently giving to the people in their lives — and they need friends who both respect and appreciate their selfless nature. To be a good friend to an ESFJ, show them that you appreciate their support, and are there to reciprocate it whenever they need it. ESFJs need people in their lives who they can vent to, share their feelings with, and rely on. If you have those bases covered, you're probably in their good books (Priebe, 2016)."

The thing about Jacobi is that she is constantly trying to help others. She doesn't cook meals, buy friends their favorite beverage when they are feeling down, or randomly text a word of encouragement to be recognized. It would be very easy for someone to miss her selfless acts because she literally always does them. So, before I go to see her, I quickly review her file and then think, "Yeah, I need to remember that she is probably going to do something to bless me or someone else and that it means a lot to her invisible self when someone recognizes that." Again, she does these things to get anything in return, but when she is acknowledged, I know it means a lot to her.

Should you tell your friends you have a file on them? That's totally up to you. Here are a few things to consider before you do:

- Some people, whether it's your friends or your wife, might/probably/most definitely will think it's weird.

- It's one more thing to add to your to-do list when it comes to maintaining your friendships.

- At some point, your friends may ask to see them. This could lead to a whole host of problems. If you have put some unappealing information about them in your file, you might want to consider this before you tell them about it or remove it before you show it to them.

I hardly ever talk about my friend files to anyone. I try to keep them up-to-date (not always perfectly) in order to develop and nurture my friendships, which is very important to me. And ... I kinda think it's fun.

*You*tilization

Take a look at your closest friends. Choose one, and create a file on them. Do you see the value in it? How do you see it helping? Is there anything about it that scares you away? For a free template to start your own friend files, and to receive a free workbook that accompanies this book, visit the website: www.broken-people.org, click "contact us" at the top, and fill in all the fields. In the comments section, type, "I'd like to receive the free workbook!"

Wanna go even deeper?

Complete a file on all your IBFs and immediate family. Then, whenever you think about it, review their file before going to spend time with them. It will make for a richer hangout experience.

IBF: When You Don't Feel Like a Friend

There were several months during this book project that I wasn't able to write a single word. I was at the spot where I was supposed to be writing about friendship yet I felt anything like a good friend. How am I supposed to write about friendship when I don't feel like I'm any good at it? Let me tell you, it ain't easy. Don't get me wrong, my friends would probably tell you that I'm a great friend. They may even go so far as to say I'm the ideal friend. So how do I reconcile feeling like I'm a big failure while my friends think I'm the bee's knees? A story of course.

Last month, my youngest son began acting out in a more violent way toward my wife and I. We reached the tipping point one night when his temper erupted. He was dropping F-bombs like they were going out of style, savagely kicked several holes in our walls, toppled his ten-gallon fish tank onto his bedroom floor, and threatened to kill me. The next day, I found a dinner plate sticking out of his wall. I left it there because I thought it'd be a good reminder of what it looks like when we don't take care of our mental health. When he threw his ten-gallon fish tank on the floor, glass and water went everywhere … including through the floor into our daughter's room below. As soon as she realized what had happened, she rushed upstairs to try to save his fish. They didn't make it. He'd only had the tank for about a week, but it had been something he had wanted for months.

The police were called, something I never thought I'd have to do with one of my children. It felt like I was in someone else's nightmare! He was taken to the emergency room in an ambulance where he and I spent the night until a room was available for him at a psychiatric hospital. He spent several days undergoing inpatient treatment for depression. My wife and I were an emotional mess. Who wouldn't be, right?

With all of that going on, I couldn't focus on my friends. I didn't feel right or even capable of thinking, let alone writing, about the topic. At the moment, we are about a week out from his most recent hospitalization and writing this is a way I'm trying to cope.

Friendship needs come and go in cycles. Having Intentional Best Friends has given me the support and peace of mind I've needed during this chaotic time in my family. They've been the people available to listen and care, night or day. These are the people I can and have turned to in my darkest hours. Wanna know how they feel about it? They feel great! This process ... this thing ... works!

I asked my friend Joe if he'd set up a GoFundMe campaign to helped us cover $6,500 in debt that resulted from several hospitalizations. It was an amazing blessing! This was just one example of the many things my friends and I do for each other.

So as I sit here typing, feeling like an awful friend, I know you've been there, too. We need to let it go. Our friends will have times like this as well. We don't want them feeling guilty for needing an extra helping of love. And when they do go through a rough patch or a field of misery, we will be there for them like they were for us. Allow your friends to love you wherever you are. That's what friends are for!

*You*tilization

Do you go through periods of insecurity with your friendships? Call or text one of your IBFs and ask, "Am I a good friend?" Listen. Believe what they say. Then write about the conversation in your journal.

Wanna go even deeper?

It is very possible that one of your friends might be struggling with feelings of inadequacy. Think about creative ways to affirm the friendships you have. Send them a letter, surprise them at home with a meaningful gift, or call them on the phone just to let them know you appreciate and love them.

IBF: What Makes Intentional Best Friends Hard?

I worked at the Grand Rapids Police Department in 1998 for less than a month. I'd gone to a community college near Detroit for three years, graduated from the Flint Regional Police Training Academy third in my class, and didn't even last a month! I'd been sworn in by the chief, but never, technically, became a fully-certified officer. Why? I was terrible at it. I was scared, lacked the necessary street smarts, and just didn't have the nerve to do the job. Thankfully, I never made it out of the training division. One day, my Lieutenant called me into his office along with the Captain who hired me. They asked for my weapon, sat me down, showed me video footage of some of my training sessions, and convinced me to throw in the towel. This is not an easy story for me to share. It's one of the more embarrassing experiences I've lived through. But just like most major life events, I've learned a lot from it.

It was hard to quit the job I'd been preparing myself to do for several years. Quitting or changing anything that's been part of your life's routine for any amount of time is tough business! When I was going through DBT with my therapist, she introduced an idea that really floored me: Sometimes it's better to let a friendship die, and possibly one day be resurrected again, than to try to keep an unhealthy relationship alive and poison the friendship beyond resuscitation. Right away, I knew of at least one friendship that I needed to let go. What I learned through this process was a lesson in gray areas. I did let the friendship go. I spent less time trying to hang out with this person. I called them less. Distance grew. They weren't included in the next year's IBF group. Interestingly enough, the friendship *never died*? Weird, right? It changed, which was what needed to happen. But it never actually stopped. It reached a healthy plateau and then continued on. And, you know what, it's been good ever since!

Complications in friendships are a normal part of life. There is a certain ebb and flow to the depth and closeness of friends. It's not wrong to acknowledge that. Life is much more difficult when we try to force something that is out of season. Not too long after I "let that friendship go," I went through some major physical and emotional battles. That friend was one of the most loving and supporting people for me and my family through some very scary stuff. We never did stop caring for each other. Just because you let a friendship go, doesn't mean it's gone. And just because a friend isn't an IBF, doesn't mean they're not a significant part of your story.

During that same year, after I sent out my IBF letters on Thanksgiving, I had one friend who felt that the commitment was more than they were capable of or willing to make. Don't get me wrong, this person cared a lot about me and my family, but they just were not able to maintain the depth of friendship I was asking for. Did it sting? Yeah, a little. But, more than anything, it impressed me. Although the friendship looks different today than it did a few years ago, we never stopped being friends. When your friends feel free and safe to share their honest feelings, even when it isn't always the most comfortable thing to do, then you know you have done a good job nurturing a healthy relationship.

If you decide to let someone know they are an IBF, there is a certain level of complexity that comes along with that decision. What happens when they're no longer an IBF? More than likely, this will happen with most, if not all, of your IBFs. Please be aware of the potential for increased anxiety that can result in the days leading up to the date you've chosen for your IBF starting day. It might be a good idea to plan an extra therapy session or two. That's what I do. Whatever you choose to do, whether it be to announce your IBFs or keep them a secret, it's important to remember that your IBFs are just a small subset of a much larger community of friends. All of your friends are important. Vital even. There is a possibility that someone might feel like a lower-class friend because they didn't make it on some special list of yours. Be mindful of this. And if it happens, if you sense jealousy or envy, take the time to sit down and talk with your friend about it. I think we both can relate to how it feels to be left out. A little understanding can go a long way.

*You*tilization

Is there a friendship you need to let go? If there is, write your fears about it in your journal. If there's not, has there ever been a relationship you think might have benefited from being let go?

Wanna go even deeper?

It's one thing to identify a friendship that needs to be let go, and another to actually do something about it. If you want to go deeper, talk to your therapist about this friendship and some of the frustrations or fears surrounding it. Share what you learned in this chapter and then, together with your therapist, come up with an action plan.

IBF: Celebrating

For Christmas this year, I bought each of my IBFs a gift. I put it in a box, wrapped it up, drove it to their home, and threw it *at* their porch. Oh yeah, and I videoed the delivery like some twisted FedEx courier's version of the COPS reality show, and sent it to them. It's fun to celebrate your friends. But it's more than just fun, it's relationship building and good for your mental health!

Why do you celebrate? What are some of the things or special days you celebrate? Birthdays, weddings, graduations, and holidays are popular, of course. What are these celebrations about? Well, your birthday is a day to celebrate you. It's the recognition of value that you have in people's lives. A wedding is a ceremony of both a legal, moral, and spiritual commitment between two, usually/hopefully, loving people. Graduations are moments to gather loved ones together to recognize the time and hard work someone has put into their education. Holidays celebrate seasons and are more universal. Each one of these celebrations is in response to a specific event that usually lasts just a few hours or less.

When we celebrate, we remember and acknowledge certain accomplishments. The event takes the thing that's being celebrated, and makes it last just a little bit longer. When you celebrate something that your friend did, you're telling them that their accomplishment was important to you too, and you are also letting them know that they are important to you. That's what you're ultimately supporting. That's the statement you're trying to make when you celebrate: that your friend is important to you (which is the most vital thing your friend can know about you).

What's an appropriate way to celebrate? Remember to remember. Remember what they have learned, what their experiences were, and what they've accomplished. Then put wheels on that memory. This means to *act on it*. Acting on it can take on a variety of forms, from a simple text message to renting a bouncy house and setting it up in their front yard. You're really only limited by the size of your budget and the constraints of your time.

Besides the obvious events, what things should we celebrate with our friends? Stop right there! *Thou shalt not should upon thyself!* Sorry. I had to. What things *can* we celebrate with our friends? Everything! You can literally stop by your friend's home today with a flock of helium balloons and a bengal tiger just because. Make a reason up. Create your own holiday. Celebrate them opening the door. You and I … we don't celebrate enough! We became adults, and all of a sudden, we think we have to take the world seriously. Sure, some things are serious, like death and taxes. But honestly, practice loving your friends through celebration, even if it doesn't make any sense.

What are some things I've celebrated? Birthdays are one of my favorite things to celebrate. "Fiddlesticks, I already celebrate birthdays." you say? But do you celebrate the mother on the birthday? Here's how I see it. Every birthday morning, my wife gets up and cooks an insanely elaborate breakfast for each of the kids and her husband (that's me). If you add all of those birthdays together, it's a pretty ridiculous number! One year, I gave my wife a card that said, "Happy 70th Birthday" while we were out celebrating one of our kids. I had done the math, adding the kids' ages together and realized my wife had done seventy birthday celebrations for our children. I'd love to say I helped, but birthdays were always her thing. And, if that's not reason enough to celebrate her, how about the fact that their mom was intimately involved in the birthing process, if you know what I mean. It's especially fun to go into those details during their birthday breakfast.

Here's an idea if you have a friend that's fond of Hostess: Let's say they had a really great day at work. Go to your local grocery store and pick up a box of those delightful Hostess Ding Dongs. Drive to their house. Go up to their door. Ring their doorbell. Drop the Ding Dongs and run like the wind! Feel free to throw a couple for good measure. This is my take on the classic Ding, Dong Ditch. And if they had a bad day? Do the same thing, but leave a note letting them know you love them.

Friends really just want to know that they are cared for, remembered, and appreciated. If your friend tells you something important, something that's happening in their life that they are excited about, write it down in their friend file *and* make a note of it in your calendar. It doesn't matter what it is. As long as it's something that's important or exciting to them. Every time you talk to a friend is a potential opportunity for celebration, so listen carefully!

Have you ever been to a celebration where it felt like it was more about the person putting the celebration on than it was about the person being celebrated? When you're celebrating a friend, make sure you check your ego at the door. Make it about them. All fingers, oohs, and aahs should be directed at them. This is actually something I struggle with a bit. When I'm feeling insecure, envious, or jealous it's really hard to get past those complicated emotions to be a blessing to your friend. If you find yourself in that situation as I have, take a second to search your heart and make sure that the motive for celebrating is truly to be a blessing to your friend. Then do your best to love and celebrate them as selflessly as possible. You will walk away feeling much better than if you hadn't.

Celebrating is actually a really great way to deal with envy. Whenever I find myself comparing what my friend has or has accomplished to what I don't have or have not accomplished, I have experienced great relief just by doubling down on the idea of celebrating. For the record, you don't have to be excited to celebrate. It helps, but it's not a necessity. Sometimes, you have to act a certain way first, and then wait for your emotions to catch up. Whatever you do, please do not leave envy undealt with.

What kind of celebration is most meaningful? There are two types of recognition I am thinking about: material and immaterial. If you have the choice between doing something tangible and doing something intangible, think about the person you are celebrating. What is important to them? Do you need to buy them a gift, or is a simple phone call or text more appropriate? Do they liked to be surprised? Or are they the type of person—like my wife- who makes out a list of exactly what they want. Oh yeah, and once you know all of this stuff, take a second to write about it in their friend file.

*You*tilization

It's time to celebrate! Think about your friends. What have they been up to? What's been going on in their lives? Pick a friend, and schedule a day to celebrate something about them before you move on to the next chapter.

Wanna go even deeper?

Set a time once a week, month, or quarter on your calendar to do something to recognize one friend. For example, if you have twelve really good friends, then each friend gets a special celebration once a year.

IBF: Creativity and Friendship

I am a rule follower. I think rules are important and designed to keep people safe and healthy. With that said, there have been times I've broken rules as a way to express love to friends. Like the time I smuggled contraband into a secure facility...

There's an inpatient psychiatric hospital near my home town that decided that food from outside the facility was no longer allowed to be brought in to patients. My friend Nathan had been a guest at this facility for several days, and if there's one thing I know about Nathan, it's that he appreciates a little harmless rule-tampering. Because I'm such a loving and creative friend, I decided that I needed do some adjusting to my morals to express creative love to my hurting friend. What did I do? I brought him a gift, of course.

I can't think of a better, safer place to develop and utilize your creativity than with your friends. So let's get those creative juices flowing. Why? Because I've found that one of the best tools I have to battle my inner demons is also inside of me—my creativity. It took me forty-one years to figure this out. Forty-one years of hating myself, thinking I was a freak, and wanting to be anyone else but me. To be fair, this self-learning has been gradually happening my entire life, and so is yours. But when major life events happen (and this has happened several times throughout my life), things just start to click ... to make sense ... life becomes a little clearer.

I've spent my life learning to embrace the uniqueness of who I am. This most recent shift, at the age of forty-one, still required a lot of intentionality and courage. This self-learning requires that on a daily basis I put my phone down, disconnect from social media, and take a dive into the deeper parts of who I am. Oh yeah, and guess what? This "diving in" to your creativity will create ripples! The kind of ripples I mentioned in an earlier chapter about journaling. The chain reaction kind.

Let's talk a bit about developing your friendships, making those relationships deeper and more fulfilling by embracing your creativity. This isn't a checklist. It's a guide, because the only way you are going to be effective doing any of this stuff is if you *You*tilize it. An important step to using creativity to build strong friendships starts with listening. When you listen well, you hear things about your friends that matter to them. Listen to the things they're saying, but also to the things they're not saying. For example, the next time you're talking with a friend and their spouse or significant other comes up, pay attention to what they say? Are they negative, constantly complaining? Or, are they always happy-go-lucky about life and their relationship? If your friend leans heavily one way or the other, ask yourself why that may be. There are a lot of potential reasons for both. Why are they telling you about the one, but not the other? This is a great opportunity to *you*tilize your friendship files. It's a lot of work, but good relationships usually are.

Another step to creatively building up your bonds of friendship is to put action into what's important to them. If you know what is important to your friends, do something to demonstrate that you understand it. Show them you're listening and that you care. This doesn't have to be a super involved process. It can be as simple as knowing they had an important meeting that day and asking them how it went. Maybe you can record a special anniversary in their friend file, and then send them a small letter or Venmo them a little cash to buy a coffee or Oreos that day. Again, listen to them. Understand them. Then act.

Does your friend have an important event coming up? What are you going to do about it? One of my friends was going to South America for four months. It was a big trip for him and his wife. He actually *quit his job* to take this trip. It obviously meant a great deal to him. As a going away "present," I went to their house late the night before they left in January, 2018, and spray painted a huge green turtle on their lawn. The lawn was completely snow covered which made a perfect canvas for spray paint art. They know how much I like turtles and this little message of endearment meant a lot to both of them. I also wrote "I like turtles" (or something as close to it as I could possibly get) in Spanish. Then I flew to my car and drove away like a scared chicken because I was freaking out that one of his neighbor's saw me lovingly vandalizing his yard and called the cops!

I have a friend that risked life and limb to bring me chocolate milk once on my birthday. As she ran through my front yard, she slipped on a "landmine" left behind by my dog, Roxy, and kissed the ground. It was so sweet—the gesture, not the "landmine." She and her kids also decorated cards for me. You don't need to spend a lot of money to do this stuff. When you establish limits on how much you can spend, or when those limits are imposed on you through that annoying budget (thank you, Dave Ramsey), it really does open up the door for your creativity—at whatever level it's at—to shine. Boundaries have a way of doing that. The main thing, as I said before, is just to remember, and then put action into what's important to them.

Don't feel creative? There's nothing wrong with not feeling creative. Most people don't realize their potential in this area, and then there are people who just don't have a creative bone in their body. Try this out, and see if it doesn't stir something up in that creativity organ in your noggin: Find a quiet place to sit. Put your phone, tablet, and laptop in **another room**. Take five deep breaths. After those five deep breaths ask yourself what you thought about while you were breathing. Pay attention to those thoughts. Then, I would like you to think about your friend. Think about the times you've spent with them, conversations you've had, stuff you know they care about. How can you connect what you know and have heard into an act of love and thoughtfulness? What can you do, remember, or say that would show them you're paying attention to them and that they matter to you? You will get distracted! Other thoughts *will* come. That's ok! Don't judge yourself for being distracted. Say "hello" to those thoughts and then get back to thinking about your friend. Did you get any ideas? I'd love to hear about them! Shoot me an email: joe@broken-people.org.

A word of caution: Pay attention to any boundaries your friends may have, and make sure that you honor them (ok, I lied, that was sixteen words). What may seem like a cute and creative idea to you, may, in fact, be annoying and aggravating to them. Luckily for me, my friend who traveled to South America never said anything to me about any boundaries in regards to people spray painting his lawn. A huge win for me! But seriously, this may seem like a little thing, but the little things add up. If your friend hates pizza, don't "celebrate" something with them by giving them a gift certificate for Little Caesars. The irony may seem funny to you, but I can assure you that it isn't a blessing to your friend.

So, back to my story about my friend Nathan. I brought him a gift. A book to be exact. I have a wide selection of books in my personal library, but there was a specific kind of book I needed for this "operation." It needed to be thick and it needed to be awful. Once I found the perfect one, I took it to my kitchen table and began my preparations. Carefully *you*tilizing a utility knife, I began carving out the middle of the book. I created a five inch by four-inch pocket, if you will, in the center of the book to store essential goodies. I then ran some Elmers glue along the inside edges of the pocket to create added support, and to keep the pages together. A person could still hold the book and quickly thumb through the pages and not notice that there was something fishy going on.

Got a rule that outside food isn't allowed? Yeah? Tell that to people at the movies when you charge a million dollars for a twelve-ounce coke … but I digress. So a book with food in it would have to do—if only I could get it through security, that was. Security ended up not being a problem (a little concerning at an inpatient facility, if you ask me). They saw me, saw the book, and let me pass. I gave the book to my friend, and he, being a person who apparently judges a book by its cover, looked at it, tried to smile, then quickly set it aside. It took a little prompting to get him to actually *look* at the book. When he finally did, the dude was smiling from ear to ear. Friendships are built and kept healthy through acts of loving-kindness. "Do" for your friends.

*You*tilization

Ok, be honest. Did you, or did you not, try the exercise on pages 261-262? If you did not, do it now. If you did, did you email me to tell me about it?

Wanna go even deeper?

Think about your friends and what they have going on in their lives right now. What friend could really use a little extra loving today? Do the exercise above with that person in mind, and then put into action what is important to them before you move on to the next chapter.

SHOULD THIS FRIENDSHIP END

Healthy friendships are great, aren't they? They make you feel alive, inspire you to live life to its fullest, and provide mutual mental, physical, spiritual, and emotional support. When my friendships are on point, my life seems a heck of a lot easier. But what about unhealthy friendships? What do we do about these relationships? That's what this whole next section is about ... dealing with complicated friendships, and hopefully giving you some ideas you can *you*tilize to live a fuller, healthier life regardless of some of its greater challenges (ie. people).

Right off the bat, I want to address the last sentence, the "regardless" comment. Do you think that life is fuller and healthier when things are only going well? It feels that way, doesn't it. In reality, challenges create opportunities for growth and personal development which are important keys to living richer and fuller lives. There are three ways I'd like you to consider dealing with difficult friendships that are the body and bones of this next section: cutting them back, cutting them off, or cutting them out.

One of the terms that gets a lot of press and will be used later is "toxic friends." Consider these definitions I found online:

Web MD says, "A toxic friendship is unsupportive, draining, unrewarding, stifling, unsatisfying, and often unequal."

Urban Dictionary: "These so-called friends backstab, gossip, lie, act selfish, use, belittle, and even manipulate and are taking more than giving back to the friendship."

I think those definitions give us a pretty good starting point as we move on to dealing with difficult people.

Cutting Back

Have you ever said to yourself about a best friend, "I can't imagine my life without this person? Like, for real, we are always going to be besties." I've felt that way with just about every close friend I've ever had. And without fail, every close friend I've ever had has, at the least, gone through a sort of cutting back. We've lost touch or just aren't as close as we once were. Often this happens naturally, but sometimes it needs to be done intentionally. Sometimes it's necessary and healthy to cut back on some friendships.

Cutting back will look different for each relationship that may need it. How do we decide when to cut back? What does cutting back even mean? Finding out when we need to cut a friendship back can be hard, so let's first decide what cutting back looks like. As I said before, it varies for each unique friendship. One of the most obvious ways to cut back is to spend less time with a person. You don't have to answer the phone every time this person calls, and you don't have to call them back the same day. What are some other things that can be cut back? Do you spend money on this person? Maybe it's a friend who has been a lunch buddy or you buy them coffee. Wait and see what happens when you purposefully decide to spend less money.

Another big way you can cut back is how you think. I'm a firm believer that we can always be cutting back on worry, which is a twisted form of thoughtfulness. In healthy or unhealthy relationships, worry is always a good thing to cut back on. Reducing the amount of time that we think about a person can be pretty hard to do, but it's possible. Consider talking to your therapist or a good friend about using mindfulness practices to think less about this person. Also, consider setting up some type of accountability with your therapist or a close friend. Have them check in regularly to see how you're doing.

Social media is constantly reminding us of things. Some good, some not. If you use social media, unfollowing someone you're cutting back on is a great way to avoid thinking about them unnecessarily. It's not harsh or rude to stop getting notifications about someone. First of all, they won't know unless you tell them. Secondly, you can still see what's going on in their life, but in a way that is more controlled and intentional.

So why do we cut back? Well, for starters, most cutting back happens naturally and usually goes unnoticed. I was just thinking about a friend I haven't spoken to in a few weeks. There's no reason—that I can think of anyway—why this happened. It just did. I still think of this guy as a good friend. The cutting back happened naturally. There are, however, good reasons why cutting back sometimes needs to happen on purpose.

One of the first reasons it may be good to cut a relationship back is that it can actually save the friendship. Remember a few chapters ago, when I talked about letting go? That's what happened with this friend. Cutting back actually saved our friendship. If you have a friend that is rubbing you the wrong way, or getting under your skin, putting some distance between you might be just what the doctor ordered. One of the biggest lessons I've learned in marriage, one of the more complicated friendships a person can have, is that when conflict happens between my wife and I, the worst thing I can do is to be around her. When we are in the middle of an argument, I want to work things out right away. I'm a problem solver. I am also terribly insecure. Both traits do me no favors in that situation. My wife is completely the opposite. She, admittedly, is a problem starter and a very secure and independent woman. When we put distance between us for a short time, we're able to clear our heads. I don't know about you, but when my emotions are in control of my mouth, as opposed to logic and reason, I can say some pretty stupid things. And when that happens, it demonstrates the exact *opposite* of what I want her to know about me: That I care more about how I feel than how she feels.

Sometimes family, work, or health situations take over our calendars, and we find we have less and less time for friends. During the COVID-19 pandemic, I haven't been able to hang out with friends as much as I'd like. Nobody has. I've tried to creatively fill in the gap, but we have all been put in the situation where it's been helpful to accept that we just can't be as close to our friends as we'd like. It just so happens that I'm writing this chapter around Christmas time, 2020, or what we call Peak Season at FedEx. This is the time of year delivery drivers disappear from their homes. At FedEx, we show up before sunrise and don't leave until long after the sun has said goodnight. I barely have time to shower. I don't go to the gym, and I almost never see my friends. But we do our best, texting and encouraging each other.

Be careful how long you decide to cut back a relationship, though. Cutting back can be healthy for a friendship, but it can also be harmful, especially if left for too long. If you're in an argument/disagreement with a friend that's lead to cutting back, it would be helpful for the people involved to agree on some kind of timeline. It may not be possible, or a good idea, to do it right away, so it's ok to wait until things calm down. When they do, give your friend some idea of when you think you'd be able to get together—with a clear head—to talk. Please keep in mind that there is usually an issue of insecurity on at least one person's part, and it is important that both people are considerate of the other person's feelings. If you feel like the other person isn't being considerate, don't retaliate. Set the standard for good behavior yourself. Treat them the way you want to be treated.

Cutting back should be the first consideration when dealing with an unhealthy relationship. But, I admit, there are times when someone needs to actually be cut off.

*You*tilization

What friend do you need to spend a little less time with, and what actions or steps do you think would be appropriate? Spend some time journaling and/or talking to your therapist about this before you take any action.

Wanna go even deeper?

Write your friend a letter telling them explicitly what problems you are having with your friendship and what you intend to do about it. What is your desired outcome? Where do you want to see your friendship in a year from now? Then fold the note and stick it in your underwear drawer. You never know when you might run across it again. You may be surprised, if it's been years, how things have turned out.

Cutting Off

Sometimes situations arise in a friendship, as I mentioned before, where a little distance is needed. Irritation and anger can get the better of us. We need to get away from a person because we don't want to say or do something we don't mean. This is not the time to cut someone off.

Just like with cutting back, deciding when to cut someone off can be tricky, so let's take a second to talk about what it is. When a friendship gets cut off, contact stops. There are no calls. No emails. No Facebook. There is no interaction. Here's the important thing: how you do this is vital.

One option to cutting someone off that is becoming more and more popular is ghosting them. According to Wikipedia, ghosting is "a practice of ceasing all communication and contact with a partner, friend, or similar individual without any apparent warning or justification, and subsequently ignoring any attempt to reach out or communicate." Please don't do this to you friend/ex-friend. Think about it. Who would you ghost? To ghost someone, you first need to have a connection with them. At one point or another, they were someone you cared about. Give this person the respect of some kind of heads up.

A civilized, albeit difficult, way to cut someone off is to talk to the person. Go figure, right? You need to be able to communicate. Communication is the cornerstone of a good relationship. That's why I created the Mental Health Scale. I can't say it enough, it's really important for friends to talk to each other. It would be very unfortunate if a misunderstanding lead to a broken relationship, but it happens all the time.

I get it. Communication is really, really hard, especially during conflict. But *you and I can do hard things!* When we tackle these issues head on, and with integrity, it only makes us better people.

The one experience I have had with cutting someone off was a long process. It happened over a period of seven years. I went through a cutting back phase with this person because they were creating a lot of extra stress in my life. After a long period of repeated selfishness, insults, and self-righteousness behavior toward my family, I decided that this friendship needed to be cut off. The cutting off started fairly naturally. During the cutting back period, and even when I began cutting him off, I was always willing for the relationship to be restored to its previous glory. He'd been one of my best friends, after all. Then one day he told me and my pastor he was convinced I was being used by the Devil to ruin their life. At that point, I knew it was over. Did I tell him I was done? Regrettably, no. In every difficult friend shituation, (which is kind of how it felt in that story), we can always look back and say, "I wish I would have done xyz better." In my situation, I felt that the cutting back had been such a long process that the cutting off was just a natural next step, not needing any type of announcement. We had already had countless conversations about this person's lifestyle choices and attitude. At some point, it just had to end. And it did.

Here are two important things I think we all should keep in mind when we cut someone off. One, don't dismiss the idea that, someday, that relationship may and can be restored. And two, try as humanly possible to live a lifestyle of forgiveness. It can be easy to cut people off when you're angry. And just as easy to hang on to that anger and have it poison your soul. Forgiveness is your response to your inner-self that says, "I'm not letting what this person did hold me captive any longer." Forgiveness doesn't say that what the person did was right, or that they don't have to deal with the consequences of their actions. It's not a universal hall pass to let people do and say whatever they want without justice. It's a vehicle for the hurt and offended to move on with life. When you forgive someone, you're setting yourself free.

How does forgiveness play out in my life? If you're anything like me, you find yourself replaying extremely painful events in your imagination. I do this all the time. I relive the pain and frustration of the moment. Why? Because in some twisted sort of way … it feels good. Just like a cigarette feels good for anxiety and getting drunk feels good when we are sad. We replay hurtful events, often recasting ourselves as someone who knows how to handle the situation better. It feels good, but what feels good isn't always good for us. Forgiveness is the hard work of allowing yourself freedom from the suffering, the rage, and the person who hurt you. It's an act of independence. When the thoughts come back into my head, as they quite often do, I acknowledge them. Then I remind myself that that situation, that person, that pain, is forgiven and that I have moved on. It really does work. This will happen for years or maybe your entire life. We relive the pain, but we also can relive the freedom of forgiveness.

What about toxic friends? What do we do about them? Here's a reality check ...aren't we all just a little bit toxic? Aren't we all a little selfish sometimes? Don't we all act in our best interests at times? I'm not excusing toxic behavior, but I am saying that just because you feel someone is toxic isn't a good enough reason, at least in my book, to end the relationship. What *is* a good, clear-cut reason to end a relationship? When it becomes dangerous. When your safety is in jeopardy, pull the plug. Get to safety!

So now that we've talked about cutting back and cutting off, it's time to consider a third option when faced with struggling relationships: cutting it out.

*You*tilization

Think about all the stuff people cut off. Things like hair, paper, budgets ... why do those things need to be cut off? Think about how this might apply to why sometimes we need to cut people off, then write your thoughts in your journal.

Wanna go even deeper?

Think about toxic people. How often have you heard someone encouraging someone else to cut off a relationship that's toxic? Journal about this. Do you think toxic people need friends? Do you think everyone is toxic like I do? Are you in a relationship that is dangerous? If you are, this is the type of relationship that needs to be cut off immediately.

Cut It Out

It takes two to tango. Have you ever heard that phrase? It is so easy to point fingers at the other person when relationships are not going well. It is equally as easy, at least it is for me, to succumb to the constant insults we hurl at ourselves in the messy battle in our heads. We can go from one extreme to the other. Cut it out.

A third option to deal with hard or unhealthy friendships is to cut it out. That's right. We need to realize that sometimes we cause problems in relationships as much as we receive the problems. If we are in the middle of a difficult situation, take the time to really sit and think about your part in it. It's easy when you're arguing to push the blame on the other person. Cut it out! Go find a spot to be quiet and consider your part.

When you're tempted, as I often am, to suck up all the blame, cut it out! You're not making the relationship better by taking ownership of issues that are not yours to own. It's not heroic to ignore the faults of other people, and it's equally not fair to always put the blame solely on the other person. Without a doubt, fault often does fall on one person more than another. Even if the fault is one hundred percent the other person's, if you don't take the time to sit, and at least reflect on any role you might have played in this, you may be missing out on a wonderful opportunity for relational growth.

We really do need to cut it out. Stop looking for easy ways to handle tough relationships. We all *go* through them. But if we do them right, we also all *grow* through them. Being invested in people, trusting people, loving people, and then letting them do it in return is one of the best decisions we can make in our life. I want to encourage you to see these things through and not cut off people so easily. Giving up is the mantra of an unhealthy mental life. Instead, embrace this idea: I can do hard things.

*You*tilization

Think about a conflict you've had with a friend recently. Ask yourself, and maybe someone who isn't emotionally invested in the conflict, is it possible that the problem may not be your friend, but you.

Wanna go even deeper?

When you have a problem at home or at work and someone confronts you about it, what happens in your head? There is an inner-dialogue that happens that affects how you deal with the stress and anxiety of that situation. Write those inner-thoughts down in your journal and share them with a close friend or therapist the next time you get together.

NOT THE END

I have mentioned three very important tools throughout this book:

A measuring tape: the Mental Health Scale

A hammer: your journal

A nail: your friends

If you've spent as much time in therapy as I have, then you know there are so many more tools to discover and use. That's one of the reasons (just one of many), why seeking professional help is so important for your mental health. You see, we have all been Broken People. Nobody goes through this life unbroken. But I also believe we are not always broken. The tools and the work we put in actual do produce healing.

There are many ways to learn, to record experiences, to pound out ideas and life lessons. There are many more connections and relationships a person can have beyond friends that help to support us and can be a part of healing our brokenness. My oldest daughter has a rustic, white dining room chair. It's one of the many purchases she made when putting together the décor for her new home. One day, my youngest daughter who lives with her, tipped the chair over, breaking the handle off the back of it. As soon as she told me what happened, I knew I could fix it. I came to the project knowing what tools to use and had a well thought out plan of execution. I'd been in this situation before.

A year after my wife and I married, the arm broke off of a very special rocking chair given to us at our wedding by her grandfather. For some reason, I thought I knew exactly what it would take to fix it. One day, while my wife was out, I got out my drill and found a couple random screws in my toolbox and went about repairing her beloved chair. When she got home, I didn't tell her what I had done. I wanted it to be a surprise. I wanted her to see how much I loved her, and that I was a guy she could count on to fix things that were broken. Later that evening, she came home and was very surprised to see that I'd" fixed" her chair. She saw the head of a screw protruding through one of the spindles in the back of the chair. She found several abandoned holes left in the wood where I struggled to force a screw through the un-predrilled wood. I was proud. She was devastated. I was hurt. She was angry. We both felt broken. Despite my best efforts, it did look awful. How could I have been so wrong? I was confident that my actions would bless my wife. I wanted to be her hero. Instead, my wife hated it, and this one story has made me somewhat of a legend in my family.

When we grow, when we try, when we fail, when we face criticism, when we act in confidence and courage, when we learn from our mistakes and celebrate our wins, we never stay the same. It's impossible! When I went to fix my daughter's chair, I brought the right tools and a few things I'd learned over the years. I pre-drilled holes through the broken piece using two different sized bits to allow for the head of the screw to sink beneath the surface of the wood, sanded the two broken surfaces to make sure they went together nicely, and used new, sturdy screws. I applied wood glue to the broken surface and gently screwed the two pieces together, sinking the head of the screw just deep enough to hide. Then I went over it with some spackle to hide the screws. All that's left for me is to get back over there to sand everything down to make it look just like new. At the moment, you can see the damage. But when it's painted, it will look like it had never been broken.

When we get hurt, when we feel broken, we don't always make the best choices. We don't always gravitate toward the healthier decisions. Maybe you've tried to rig some kind of personal treatment together without a lot of experience or guidance from people who know better or who've been there. Maybe you did something like I did with my wife's rocking chair, taking a tool I'd never really used before and finding some random screws lying around thinking they would do the job; trying to force solutions into the broken pieces, hoping to make everything better. You may even feel slightly better and proud of your accomplishment when you do. And why shouldn't you? We are all on a path of discovery. We make the best choices we can with the life experience we have, then realize, hopefully, that there are better options.

As you *you*tilize these helpful tools and go all the way through the healing process, it can appear to others around you that you had never been broken before, because it looks like you have it all together. You know you don't. You know all the work it took to heal. You see the small cracks. That is why it is so important that you don't pretend you were never broken. People need to know that they are not alone and that there is hope. Everyone needs to hear that *broken doesn't mean forever.*

RECOMMENDED BOOKS

Subject	Book
Boundaries	*Boundaries* by Dr. Henry Cloud & John Townsend
Courage	*Rising Strong* by Brené Brown
Faith	*Mere Christianity* by C.S. Lewis
Fear	*Fearless* by Max Lucado
Forgiveness	*The Book of Forgiveness* by Desmond Tutu
Gratitude	*One Thousand Awesome Gifts* by Ann Voskamp
Habits	*The Power of Habit* by Charles Duhigg
Happiness	*The Happiness Equation* by Neil Pasricha
Life Lessons	*How to Win Friends and Influence People* by Dale Carnegie
Love	*The Five Love Languages* by Gary Chapman
	Love Does by Bob Goff

BROKEN LIKE ME

Parenting Kids	*How to be a Hero to your Kids* by Josh McDowell & Dick Day
Parenting Teens	*Have a New Teenager by Friday* by Kevin Leman
Understanding your Why	*Start With Why* by Simon Sinek

ACKNOWLEDGMENTS

Hundreds of people have played a vital role in the formation of this project. The idea and heart behind Broken People has countless origins. It's a culmination of life lessons and the great people God has seen fit to put in my path. My friends Ronnie and Jan Kirkconnell, the late James Hoag, and Shawn Richter who were the original group of Broken People who helped me build a seventeen-foot beer bottle for Art Prize, 2016. Nathan Beals, whose death and life inspired me to heal, his sister Annie Hightower who is constantly encouraging me, and Clarkston Morgan, who inspired me to do more than just write a book, but to start a movement.

Several people have either been to my house to help discuss and critique the concepts and structure of this book or have been a tremendous help via our beloved technology: David and Carol Tiesma, Mike and Breanne Keller, Dan and Megan Deweerd, Joseph Joslin, Jeff and Jacobi Warners, Adam Lipscomb, Carol Hines, Amanda Duncan, Amanda Waldron, Dana Sullivan, Pamela Squire, Rebecca Zaagman, and Caleb Roede. I couldn't have made it here without you!

Nathan Sweeney, Sarah Nichols, Joe Joslin, and Rebecca Reid, your editing skills are top notch. Thanks for giving so much love and time to this project.

Jen Henderson, formatting a book isn't anything I ever knew existed prior to this project! You made this very scary venture, with all its unknowns, come to life. Thank you.

To NAMI Kent County, thank you for adopting me into the fray and letting me serve with you. Your mission and people are amazing!

To the Broken People Leadership Team: Donda Cox, Johnna Paraiso, and Doug Roede. Thank you for your support and effective leadership.

To my friends at City Life Church in Grand Rapids, MI. Thank you for giving me a place to grow and heal from my brokenness.

To my wonderful family: Melissa, Olivia, Hannah, Zackary, and David. It has been quite the few years, hasn't it? You're all my favorite!

And finally, to God the Father, Jesus Christ his son, and his Holy Spirit. I don't understand you, but I trust you. I wouldn't be the person I am today if not for your grace and strength. I love you more than my life. Thank you for your faithfulness to your beloved.

ABOUT THE AUTHOR

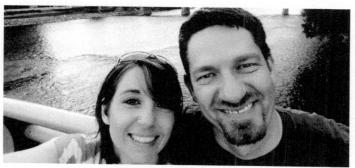

Joseph (and wife Melissa) Reid,
Grand Rapids, MI

I'm really excited about writing this part because I can pretty much say whatever I want about myself and my editor will just have to find a way to live with it! So what do I want you to know about me? I love Jesus! I really do think there is something unique and precious about his story and love for the world. It has forever changed my life.

I actually like Southern tea better than chocolate milk, but it is so hard to find a place that serves it just the way I like it. I am a graduate from several educational programs: Henry Ford Community College (1996) with an Associates in Science, Flint Regional Police Academy (1997), Global University around (2003-ish), and Liberty

University (2017) with a Bachelors in Interdisciplinary Studies. I am passionate about loving people, but it also wears me out. Hence all the talk about boundaries. I would really like to hear from you and what you thought about my book. Shoot me an email: joe@broken-people.org.

And for all those people who know me very well and have been waiting, just waiting for me to say something about turtles … you know I like 'em.

CAN YOU HELP?

Thank You for Reading My Book!

I really appreciate all of your feedback,
and I love hearing what you have to say.

I need your input to make the next version
of this book and my future books better.

Please leave me an honest review on Amazon
letting me know what you thought of the book.

Thanks so much!

Joseph Reid

REFERENCES

Ando, R. and Sakamoto, A. (2008). The effect of cyber-friends on loneliness and social anxiety: Differences between high and low self-evaluated physical attractiveness groups. Computers in Human Behavior. 24. 993-1009.

Caruso, G. (March 2013). Journaling helps woman lose half her body weight. CNN. Retrieved from: https://www.cnn.com/2013/03/01/health/journaling-weight-loss/index.html.

Gross. E. L. How journaling can help you succeed at work. monster.com. Retrieved from: https://www.monster.com/career-advice/article/journalingideas-0617

Hamm, T. (Feb 2018). How daily journaling can improve your financial life. U.S. News and World Report. Retrieved from: https://money.usnews.com/money/blogs/my-money/articles/2018-02-27/howdaily-journaling-can-help-improve-your-financial-life

How to make a nature journal. (November, 2020). How to Make a nature journal. WikiHow.com Retrieved from: https://www.wikihow.com/Make-a-Nature-Journal#References

Lennon, J. & McCartney, P. (1964). A Hard Day's Night. *A Hard Day's Night*. Parlophone [UK]. Capitol [US].

Murray, Bridget. (June 2002). Writing To Heal. American Psychological Association. Vol 33. No. 6. Retrieved from: https://www.apa.org/monitor/jun02/writing

Philip M. Ullrich, M.A. and Susan K. Lutgendorf, Ph.D. (2002). Journaling About Stressful Events: Effects of Cognitive Processing and Emotional Expression. Annals of Behavioral Medicine. 24(3). 244-250

Priebe, Hiede. (2016, January 28). How to be a good friend to each Meyers-Briggs Personality Type. Thought Catalog. Retrieved from https://thoughtcatalog.com/heidi-priebe/2016/01/how-to-be-a-good-friend-to-each-myers-briggs-personality-type/

Prime Minister's Office. Department of Digital, Culture, Media & Sport. Office for Civil Society. The Rt Hon Teresa May MP. (October 2018). PM launches government's first loneliness strategy. [Press Release] Retrieved from: https://www.gov.uk/government/news/pm-launches-governments-first-loneliness-strategy

Psychosocial Intervention: Definition & Examples. (2017, October 15). Retrieved from https://study.com/academy/lesson/psychosocial-intervention-definition-examples.html.

Scott,Vann B.,,Jr, Robare, R. D., Raines, D. B., Konwinski, S. J. M., Chanin, J. A., & Tolley, R. S. (2003). Emotive writing moderates the relationship between mood awareness and athletic performance in collegiate tennis players. North American Journal of Psychology, 5(2), 311-324. Retrieved from http://ezproxy.liberty.edu/login?url=https://search-proquest.com.ezproxy.liberty.edu/docview/197982635?accountid=12085

Made in the USA
Monee, IL
01 June 2021